Biomedical Instrumentation

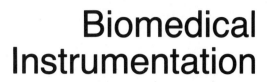

Biomedical Instrumentation

MARVIN D. WEISS

CHILTON BOOK COMPANY

PHILADELPHIA • NEW YORK • LONDON

Copyright © 1973 by Marvin D. Weiss
First Edition   All Rights Reserved
Published in Philadelphia by Chilton Book Company
and simultaneously in Ontario, Canada,
by Thomas Nelson & Sons, Ltd.

Library of Congress Cataloging in Publication Data

Weiss, Marvin D
    Biomedical instrumentation.

    Bibliography: p.
    1.   Medical instruments and apparatus.   2.   Biomedical
engineering.   I.   Title.   [DNLM: 1.   Biomedical
engineering.   QT   34   W399b   1973]
R856.W45   574'.028   72–11805
ISBN 0–8019–5688–9

Designed by Donald Cooke

Manufactured in the United States of America

Dedicated to
My Students
Who Are My Teachers

Preface

BIOMEDICAL INSTRUMENTATION is derived from branches of diverse disciplines. It borrows from physics, chemistry, biology, and medical science. It uses data from electrical, mechanical, and chemical engineering and from instrumentation technology. It also uses information derived from physiology, thermodynamics, hydraulics, systems engineering, and simulation.

To master the subject, the student must have a good working knowledge of these basic disciplines. Since such knowledge is not presented in any currently available text, it became necessary here to provide the underlying principles of these disciplines. The teacher may use the book to provide background for his lectures. The independent researcher may find the material useful in carrying his research over a difficult point.

Historically, cybernetics has served to draw together the biological scientist and the engineering technologist. We draw upon this discipline to help explain the merging of science and technology in the study of biological or instrumentation systems. Communication and control in biological systems can be understood in terms of the techniques of communication and control of electronic systems. The techniques of systems analysis and simulation help to explain them both. Thus, the sciences are interwoven with technology, using cybernetics as part of the interlocking pattern.

Chapter 1 outlines the general scope of the book, and provides a summary of the tools required to understand metrology, physiology, and simulation. Metrology, the science of instrumentation, provides the basis for preparing and evaluating studies of measuring instruments. Physiology, the study of the functioning of the human body, provides the basis for understanding the sources and applications of medical instrumentation. Simulation, the study of the interaction of variables, provides the basis for the nonmathematical use of mathematical principles in the analysis of instrumentation and physiological systems.

Chapters 2 and 3 are concerned with the principles of electronics and their application to measuring systems. The principles of electronics and their combining into operating circuits are used to explain measuring systems of transducers, bridges, amplifiers, and display and recording equipment. This information, familiar enough to the practicing engineer, should prove invaluable as background for the medical and life science practitioner.

Chapter 4 furnishes the engineer and physicist with information parallel to that furnished the biologist in the previous chapters, i.e., an introduction to a different discipline. Elementary physiology is presented from an advanced standpoint. The elementary principles of the cell, nervous system, circulatory system and the control of body fluids are presented, together with the block diagrams of the biophysical systems involved.

Chapters 5 and 6 present material new to both life science and control engineering students. In the past 20 years analysis instrumentation has emerged as an interdisciplinary area in which both the chemist and physicist have contributed to the measurement of the chemical composition of a dynamic system. Although developed for industrial process control, the principles have been applied to the development of biomedical instrumentation for monitoring and diagnosis. Electrochemical principles of analysis are discussed in Chapter 5 and electromagnetic radiation methods of analysis in Chapter 6.

Chapter 7 is the first chapter devoted to medical practice. The previous chapters have provided us with the tools required to understand the equipment being developed to monitor hospitalized patients. A survey of the field is presented, emphasizing the applicability of principles examined in previous chapters. We learn how these principles are applied to hospital sensors, patient monitors and central display stations. With our background in electronics, we can clearly see the hazards of allowing electrical equipment to be placed in the hands of unskilled hospital personnel.

Chapter 8 describes and explains the diagnostic equipment used by the physician. The stethoscope and sphygmomanometer (blood pressure cuff), as well as some of the newer instruments (respiratory gas analyzers, kidney function analyzers, phonocardiographs and automatic blood analyzers) are discussed at length.

Chapter 9 surveys the research laboratory for the more recent developments in medical instrumentation. In Chapter 10 we study the computer to find out how its high-speed computation and analytical features expedite the mass of data produced by the new instruments. Finally, Chapter 10 discusses some of the systems that have been proposed for biomedical instrumentation. The analysis of normal biological mechanisms is used for the explanation and control of disease states as well as for the maintenance of health.

A glossary defines engineering terms for the medical student and medical terms for the engineering student. The biologist may be disturbed because we have used layman's language to describe his field, and the engineer may be equally exercised because we have kept the terms from his field on an elementary level. However, each will be mollified because we have avoided technological jargon in a field not his own.

With this knowledge of circuit and systems analysis and instrumentation, the biomedical practitioner will be able to understand the equipment he is expected to use; provide emergency services and direct the serviceman to the problem area when difficulties with equipment arise; understand the specifications for proposed equipment and write specifications that will provide the proper equipment for the use intended; evaluate proposed and actual equipment for proper performance; and maintain safety in the laboratory, clinic, operating room, and hospital.

If a majority of these goals is achieved, this textbook will have served its purpose.

MARVIN D. WEISS
Valparaiso, Indiana

Contents

.

Biomedical Instrumentation

Chapter 1

Introduction to Biomedical Instrumentation

BIOLOGICAL SYSTEMS AND CYBERNETICS

During World War II it was the custom of a group of scientists of varied backgrounds to meet at the Harvard Medical School for lunch, and to discuss their respective vocations. They soon found that when a physiologist discussed "homeostasis," he meant the same thing that an electrical engineer meant when he said "servomechanism." Feedback is the universal principle of nature that governs the behavior of both living and nonliving systems. In this group Norbert Wiener coined the word *Cybernetics* to include "communication and control in man and in machine."

The study of biological systems is but another branch of systems theory. The physiologist who studies the function of living systems finds that he is studying the physics and chemistry of the components of the system, expressing them in mathematical form, and building a mathematical model of his biological system. The control of fluids in the body, or the history of an electronic signal through the myocardium of the heart, requires the application of principles similar to those found in the study of an automated plant for the production of milk bottles. Cybernetics, the feedback principle applied to the relationship between the parts of a system, provides the means of understanding the whole, based on measurements of the parts.

In a popular text on medical physiology, the first chapter is called "Functional Organization of the Human Body and Control of the 'Internal Environment,'" even as an electrical engineering text might have a chapter entitled "Functional Organization of a Power Plant and Control of its Internal Environment." In one case we are dealing with *homeostasis*, the ability of a living organism to control its internal environment; in the other case we are dealing with *feedback control*, the ability of a system to remain within control by measuring one of its variables and adjusting another variable in a manner that will reduce its deviation from the desired state.

PHYSIOLOGY

Physiology is the study of the functioning of living organisms. Human physiology (with which we shall be mainly concerned) is an attempt to define by principles of physics and chemistry the mechanisms by which human beings function. Starting with the chemical reactions that occur in the cells, the process whereby oxygen and food are brought to the cells and waste products are eliminated, the study builds a hierarchy of systems of increasing complexity until ultimately we have the entire man, with his hunger and thirst, his desire for love and understanding, his need for a favorable environment, his automatic adjustment when he must cope with unfavorable surroundings, and his physicochemical mechanisms underlying the principal functions of the body.

Instrumentation makes it possible for us not only to observe this system in operation without too much disturbance of the function, but also to detect malfunctions and to help repair them. Much as an alarm in the control center of a ship signals "high temperature in the boiler room," a biomedical sensor informs the physician that irregularities in the blood pressure pattern are occurring which indicate incipient disease.

Physiology, which we may call the systems analysis of the entire organism, is subdivided into branches which may be called "systems analysis of the subsystems." Thus, neurophysiology deals with the systems analysis of the nervous system, i.e., the communications system of the organism. How are nervous signals transmitted? How does the brain operate? How do we convert a color into an image in the brain? Why do we react quickly to a hot surface by a "reflex action" yet react not at all to strong stimuli which do not threaten the safety of the organism?

The circulatory system contains a pump (the heart), which moves a fluid through myriad pathways in the organism to bathe every cell in that system. It provides the amounts of food required by the cells and removes the waste products. It also carries hormones and endocrine fluids, which command the cells to perform certain operations required for the health or survival of the organism. Since many body processes are regulated by osmosis through cell membranes, it is essential that the average body water concentration remain within narrow limits. When the lower moisture limit is approached, an *osmoreceptor* informs the brain, which in turn causes the secretion of antidiuretic hormone (ADH), which when carried by the blood to the kidneys slows the removal of water from the body until more water is imbibed.

The respiratory system provides the oxygen needed for continued survival. Chemoreceptors are continuously monitoring the carbon dioxide and oxygen levels and pH (acidity-alkalinity) of the blood, which are representative of those of the tissues of the body. If the carbon dioxide level increases, or the oxygen level or pH decreases, the inspiratory center is commanded to breathe more, bringing more air into the lungs and transmitting more oxygen to the tissues. When prolonged exercise causes depletion of available oxygen, the body by a complex chemical chain is able to accumulate an "oxygen debt." Adenosine triphosphate (ATP), which supplies energy, is converted to adenosine diphosphate (ADP). Later, after the exercise is completed, deep breathing for a prolonged period provides the oxygen needed to reconvert ADP to ATP.

The digestive system is a chemical factory that grinds and breaks down food products into the chemical building blocks that the cells need to construct additional tissue, or to react with oxygen to produce energy, or to form the magical helix of DNA. Contained in the nuclei of all cells, DNA appears to be the molecule which controls the functioning of the cell.

Finally, we have the cell itself, the basic component of our living system. Every cell at rest has electrical properties similar to every other cell. When the cell starts functioning, its electrical properties change. By means of microelectrodes we can determine that the outside of a cell is 65 millivolts (mv.) higher in potential than the inside of the cell (Table 1.1). We can measure a high concentration of sodium outside the cell (145 milliequivalents per liter) and a high concentration of potassium inside the cell (155 milliequivalents per liter).

TABLE 1.1 TYPICAL CELL PROPERTIES

(a) Ion Concentration

	Inside Cell	Outside Cell
Potassium	155 meq./L.	4 meq./L.
Sodium	12 meq./L.	145 meq./L.
Chloride	5 meq./L.	105 meq./L.

(b) Membrane Properties

Membrane Thickness	10 mμ
Potential Difference	65 mv.
Resistance	1000–10,000 ohms/cm.
Capacitance	1 micro farad
Dielectric Constant	5
Phase Angle	75°

THE ANATOMY OF THE CELL

The cell (Figure 1.1) is transparent but its ultrastructure becomes visible under the electron microscope (EM) when stained with various dyes. Inside the cell the EM picks out *organelles* (internal organs of the cell), each with a specific function. The *nucleus* contains both DNA and RNA, which have been shown to be the information carriers of the cell. The small *nucleolus* within the nucleus is richer in DNA than in RNA and is believed to be the storage area of proteins to be synthesized. In the cytoplasm surrounding the nucleus the three organelles shown are the *mitochondria*, the *endoplasmic reticulum*, and the *centrosome*.

The mitochondria comprise the energy factory of the cell. When nutrients and oxygen enter the organelle, the enzyme which is present causes a chemical reaction which produces ATP. The ATP then roams through the cell, releasing its energy wherever it may be needed. The endoplasmic reticulum, the chemical factory of the cell, forms a series of small canals. Here special secretions are made, as required. Glycogen (an inactive form of glucose) is stored in the

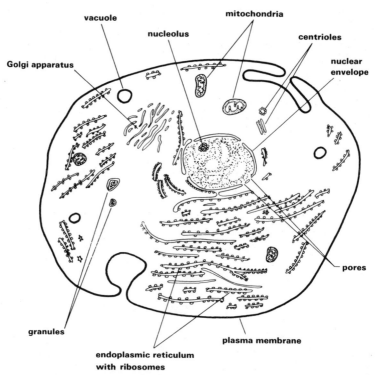

Figure 1.1 Ultrastructure of typical animal cell. (From J. Awapara *Introduction to Biological Chemistry* © 1968. By permission of Prentice-Hall, Englewood Cliffs, N.J.)

canals. Enzymes in this structure convert glucose to glycogen for storage and back to glucose when energy is needed. The *centrosome* participates in the reproduction of the cell. When cell division (mitosis) is about to take place, the centrosome splits into two asters which move to separate parts of the cell and form the basis for the formation of two nuclei from the single nucleus now in the cell, each nucleus containing the exact chromosome-gene-DNA structure of the existing nucleus.

THE SCIENCE OF INSTRUMENTATION

Lord Kelvin once said: "When you can measure what you are studying, and express it in numbers, you have advanced to the stage of science." Thus, measurement converts an art to a science. The medical arts are going through just such a transformation today, and the science of instrumentation is performing that conversion.

The science of instrumentation is composed of many parts, one of which, metrology, is concerned with the accuracy of measurement. No measurement is ever exact, but statistics supplies us with a tool to specify exactly how exact our measurement may be. The precision of a measurement is the root-mean-square deviation of the replicate of that measurement. Given the series of blood pressure measurements 120, 122, 125, 118, and 115, we add them and divide by their number (5) to obtain their average (120). This is our estimate of the *expected value* of the measurement. But how precise is this estimate? We now calculate the deviation of each measurement from the average, square the deviation, add these squares, divide by n − 1, and take the square root to obtain the root-mean-square deviation of 3.80, which is our measure of precision. Precision is not the whole story in the determination of accuracy, however. Our scale may have been moved 1 mm. from its correct position. Hence, the true blood pressure may be 119 rather than 120. To determine the correct position of the scale we need to standardize our instrument.

Accuracy then is the error caused by random events (precision) plus

EXAMPLE 1 ROOT-MEAN-SQUARE CALCULATION OF PRECISION

Measurement	−	Average	=	Deviation	(Deviation)^2
120	−	120	=	0	0
122	−	120	=	2	4
125	−	120	=	5	25
118	−	120	=	−2	4
115	−	120	=	−5	25
600					58

Sum ÷ number of measurements (n) = 600 ÷ 5   /4   14.5 = variance
= 120 (average)

root-mean-square deviation = $\sqrt{14.5}$ = 3.80

the error caused by deviation from a standard. It is usually expressed in per cent, e.g., total per cent error $= \dfrac{3.80 + 1.00}{200} \times 100 = 2.40\%$ (if 200 were the range of our instrument). We say that the accuracy of the measurement was 2.4% (when we really mean that the error was 2.4%).

ACCURACY VS PRECISION

Precision is defined as a statistic which represents the reproducibility of a measurement. *Accuracy* is defined as the difference between the measured value and the true value of a measurement. To establish the true value of a measurement, we need a *standard*. Then we can calibrate our measuring instrument against that standard to determine the accuracy of our measurement.

We have demonstrated the procedure for obtaining the precision of our measurement; now let us examine a procedure for obtaining the accuracy by calibration against a standard.

EXAMPLE 2   CALIBRATION OF A PRESSURE GAUGE AGAINST A STANDARD

A sphygmomanometer cuff is connected both to a pressure gauge and to an accurately calibrated manometer (calibrated with an accuracy of 0.01 mm. Hg). The cuff is mounted on an iron pipe, and the pressure bulb squeezed to various levels of pressure. The following readings were recorded:

Manometer	0.00	10.00	20.00	35.00	50.00	70.00	90.00
Pressure gauge	0.00	9.50	19.45	33.35	49.85	69.90	88.70
Error	0.00	−0.50	−0.55	−1.65	−0.15	−0.10	−1.30

When making the measurement, one subtracts the error for that reading to obtain the true value of the measurement.

OTHER STATISTICS OF MEASUREMENT

In addition to accuracy and precision, the measurement specialist is concerned with the sensitivity and reliability of a measurement. The sensitivity is the change in output of an instrument divided by the change in the input variable. How many divisions will a pressure gauge needle move for a 1 mm. change in the pressure in the sphygmomanometer cuff?

Reliability has also come to have a specific mathematical meaning. Defined in terms of *mean time between failure* (MTBF), one tests samples of components until they all fail. Statistics are used to calculate the mean and the standard deviation of the failure time. Accelerated testing procedures have been developed, so that one does not have to wait ten years to find that this is the mean time between failures. For example, if one were to make 20 blood pressure measurements a day for 300 working days per year, one would perform 6000 measurements per year. In an accelerated test, if one found that the equipment failed after an average of 60,000 tests, one could estimate a ten-year mean time between failures. The actual procedure involves tables, calculated on statistical principles, and provides more reliable extrapolated figures.

STANDARDS OF MEASUREMENT

The accuracy of all measurements in the United States is traceable to the standards maintained by the National Bureau of Standards Laboratory near Washington, D.C. These standards are derived in turn from the international standards maintained at the International Standards Laboratory located at Sèvres, France. Because of the growing demand for higher accuracy in our standards, current standards are much more accurate than when they were originally established, or even than they were ten years ago. New primary standards have been established for length and time, based on reliable atomic phenomena (in 1960 for length, and in 1964 for time).

The National Bureau of Standards (NBS) has several grades of standards, such as primary standards, secondary standards, derived standards, and international standards. The first three are different from the international primary standards preserved at Sèvres, France, as we shall soon see.

Primary standards are carefully preserved standards of mass, length, and time, used as a reference to establish the accuracy of secondary standards and of derived standards. The NBS primary standard is used to calibrate secondary standards, which are used by local standards laboratories to calibrate their primary standards, from which they can calibrate the secondary standards used in their laboratories. Just as the NBS primary standard is related to the international primary standard at Sèvres, so the local laboratory standards of the large manufacturing companies and of the various services are related by calibration to the primary standard at NBS. The local laboratories say their standards are traceable to the National Primary Standard.

The secondary standards are used for calibrating other pieces of measuring equipment, such as gauge blocks in machine shops, standard weights for laboratory balances, and scales calibrated by local weight and measures inspectors. Derived standards are calibrated by a combination of secondary standards, so that there is a standard for the acceleration of gravity, G, for the standard height at sea level, and for the pressure of a standard atmosphere.

International standards have been established recently for electrical quantities, instead of having them derived from the fundamental standards of mass, length, and time. There are three international standards, the volt, ohm, and temperature scale. The international volt is based on a set of standard cells also maintained at Sèvres. We have our NBS set of standard cells which we compare with those at Sèvres. Similarly, we have a set of resistance coils to establish the national standard of the ohm, based on the set of coils at Sèvres that establishes the international ohm. The international temperature scale is based on the triple point of water and the melting point of several pure materials, and a secondary standard over certain regions based on a resistance thermometer, a standard platinum thermocouple, and a radiation pyrometer.

NEW INTERNATIONAL STANDARDS

Until 1960, the international standard of length was a closely guarded platinum-iridium bar upon which was scratched the length of a meter. The new international standard established in 1960 is the wavelength of the light emitted by a lamp containing krypton 86. The meter is now defined as 1,650,763.73 wavelengths of this orange-red light.

In October 1964, the new international standard of time was established, based on the period of a cesium 133 clock, which is $1/9{,}192{,}631{,}770.0$ of a second. Previously, the second was defined as $1/86{,}400$ of a mean solar day.

The only international standard that has survived the atomic age is that for mass. It is a highly polished cylinder of platinum-iridium which represents the mass of 1 kilogram (Kg.). To preserve the integrity of this standard, it has been used only twice in the past 90 years—once in 1889, and once in 1946.

The International Temperature Scale, adopted in 1927 and revised in 1948, extends from the oxygen point (b.p. = $-182.970°C$) to the gold point (f.p. = $1063.0°C$). Four intermediate points are given: the triple point of water, $0.01°C$; the boiling point of steam, $100°C$; the boiling point of sulphur, $444.600°C$; and the freezing point of silver, $960.8°C$. The triple point of water is the point at which water, ice, and water vapor exist in equilibrium. Below the oxygen point, a set of secondary standards is maintained at NBS: a platinum resistance capsule to $10°$ Kelvin (°K); a gas thermometer from $10°K$ to $4°K$; the vapor pressure of helium from $4.2°K$ to $1°K$. Below $1°K$ the magnetic properties of paramagnetic salts are used, but each decimal place below $1°K$ becomes infinitely more difficult to measure.

Other secondary standards are provided for interpolation between the International Temperature Standards. A platinum-resistance thermometer is the standard from the oxygen point to the antimony point (f.p. = $630.5°C$); a platinum/platinum-rhodium thermocouple is the standard from the antimony point to the gold point; and an optical pyrometer is the standard above $1063°C$, the gold point, its reading calibrated by the theoretical laws of radiation pyrometry. (For more details see Chapter 3.)

ELECTRICAL STANDARDS

Electrical standards are no longer derived by reference to the primary standards of mass, length, and time. They are determined from the national standards of resistance and voltage. The resistance standard consists of ten one-ohm coils, and the voltage standard consists of a set of standard cells. (See Potentiometry, Chapter 5.) Secondary standards of all sizes of resistance are established in terms of the ten coils. There are 40 standard cells for voltage established at NBS, accurate to a few parts in ten million.

Other electrical measurements such as current, capacitance, inductance, and magnetic field strength are established by reference to the standards just enumerated, to an accuracy of 10 parts per million.

TRANSDUCERS

The object of our instrument is to obtain information from a biological system. Nature provides this information in terms of temperature, blood pressure, a sound, or a chemical composition. We want to be able to read the value of this variable on a meter, record it on a chart, or display it on an oscilloscope. The meter, the chart, or the oscilloscope, however, is activated by an electrical signal, a current, or a voltage. Hence, we require a device that will convert the natural variable to an electrical variable. Such a device is called a *transducer*.

The electrical transducer we shall use converts our biological signal to an electrical signal. There are transducers that convert measured variables to mechanical (displacement or pressure), pneumatic, or hydraulic signals. A thermometer and a sphygmomanometer are examples of these. The thermometer transduces a temperature to a displacement of the mercury column. The sphygmomanometer converts a pressure to a length displacement of the column of mercury, or the pressure gauge used for display to an angular displacement.

The transducer usually has three stages including sensor, modifier, and transmitter. The sensor responds to the variable being measured and converts it to a useful (electrical?) signal. The modifier conditions and amplifies the signal so that it can be utilized. The transmitter then sends the signal to a display unit, which may be a meter or a cathode ray tube nearby, or a digital printer some distance away.

ANALYSIS INSTRUMENTATION

For analytical measurements determined inside the organism, or in clinical laboratories, a large number of continuous and discrete sample analyzers have been developed by process control laboratory personnel in the chemical and petroleum industries. Termed *analysis instrumentation,* these devices have been used in industrial plants since about 1950 for continuous monitoring of process parameters. *Analytical instruments,* on the other hand, are pieces of laboratory equipment that have been used by chemists for instrumental methods of analysis of samples brought to the laboratory from on-stream operations in the plant. Evaluation of final product quality and compliance of raw materials to specification are also made here.

Analytical measurements will be divided in this discussion into two parts: physical measurements and electrochemical methods. Physical measurements are obtained by observing the interaction of electromagnetic radiation with the sample. Each element and compound has specific absorption properties for parts of the electromagnetic spectrum, and the "fingerprints" of the molecules present in a sample may be obtained by the use of the proper range of radiation. Each range has its own energy sources, its own difficulties in transmission through samples and carrier cells, and its own unique detection device. These factors will be discussed in greater detail in Chapter 5.

The second subdivision of analysis instrumentation is electrochemical measurements. By inserting electrodes into proper parts of the body and providing proper currents or voltages, one may measure oxygen level; pH (acid-base condition); sodium, potassium, and calcium concentrations; as well as concentrations of various other specific ions. Polarography or voltammetry—the relationship of voltage to current in certain solutions—has played a major role in clinical work in European hospitals. It is hoped that the information presented in Chapter 4 will provide the impetus for the growth of both in vivo and in vitro electrochemical methods in the United States.

SIMULATION OF BIOLOGICAL SYSTEMS

Since 1955 it has been accepted that physical, chemical, and biological processes can be simulated by electrical circuits. Later in this discussion we shall show how the analog and digital computer can be used in the study of biological processes. Models will be developed, based on information supplied by instrumentation, that will aid in the diagnosis of biological malfunctions, or in the understanding of biological systems as defined by our measurements.

Electrical parameters such as those already discussed under transducers, i.e., resistance, capacitance, and inductance, have their physical analogies in mechanical, chemical, fluid, and thermal systems. Since the body is composed of mechanical systems as exemplified by muscle and bone; chemical systems as in the cells, blood, lymph, and other fluids; fluid flow in the circulatory system; a thermal control system, as well as the heart as a powerful pump, and the digestive system as a chemical factory, all these systems must be analogous to some electrical phenomenon which can be simulated on proper computers to explain the functional behavior of the components, subsystems, and systems of the parts as well as of the whole.

As awareness of the techniques pervades the field, both engineers and medical specialists have used the technique of simulation to help explain physiological phenomena.

Before we can use electrical phenomena to define the characteristics of biomedical systems, we need to understand the electronic phenomena presented in the next chapter. Before taking up that discussion, let us look first at the tool by which systems can be represented: the block diagram.

PRINCIPLES OF SIMULATION

THE BLOCK DIAGRAM

A block diagram is a pictorial representation of the structure of a system. It represents the logical pattern of physical and mechanical elements which interact between input and output of a system. Each block in the diagram represents an element or a component of the system. The transfer function is the mathematical representation of output divided by input. If G is a transfer function, x is the input, and y is the output, then

$$G = y/x$$

The block which corresponds to this equation is shown in Figure 1.2.

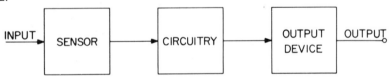

Figure 1.2 Block diagram of input-output. (From S. E. Summer *Electronic Sensing Controls*. Philadelphia: Chilton, 1969.)

G can be any mathematical relationship except addition or subtraction. (For the latter procedures the special symbol shown in Figure 1.3, the circle, is used.)

Figure 1.3 Addition-subtraction element. (From B. G. Lipták (ed.) *Instrument Engineers' Handbook* (Vol. II). Philadelphia: Chilton, 1970.)

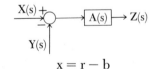

$$x = r - b$$

Note that small letters are used on the lines and capital letters in the block. The small letters represent variables, e.g., r and b could represent two temperatures:

$$r = \text{the desired temperature set on a thermostat,}$$

and

$$b = \text{the actual temperature of the room.}$$

Then,

$$y = r - b$$

where y would be the difference between the desired temperature and the actual temperature (the error in the temperature). Our thermostat might function in a manner so that when this error was five degrees the heater would be activated.

G, on the other hand, represents a functional relationship. When the thermostat goes on, the temperature of the room rises in a measurable manner. G would represent the mathematical equation which connects the functioning increase of the temperature of the room with the physical situation that the thermostat has closed.

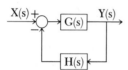

Figure 1.4 Input-comparator section of block. (From B. G. Lipták (ed.) *Instrument Engineers' Handbook* (Vol. II). Philadelphia: Chilton, 1970.)

Combining the block with the circle we have a representation (Figure 1.4) of what happens as the temperature of the room (b) changes. In Figure 1.4 since $G = y/x$, $y = Gx$, but $x = r - b$. Therefore $y = G(r - b)$. If the temperature of the room is measured by a bulb with transfer function H, we can close the loop (Figure 1.5).

We have introduced a new symbol—the take-off point—which makes it possible to measure y without disturbing y. Although the variable we take off is y, the value emerging from the point is also y, so that loss in y occurs when we measure it. This is a representation of the ideal measuring condition in which we do not disturb the variable when we measure it. (Philosophically, this condition rarely occurs exactly, but the disturbance we produce in making our measurement must be insignificant in reference to the size of the variable we measure. Hence, if we measure the temperature of a room, some heat must go into the bulb. In measuring a temperature of 70°F, the heat removed by the bulb may decrease the temperature of the room by 0.001°F. Such disturbances are disregarded in the normal course of measuring.) The closed loop produced in Figure 1.5 is known as the canonical form of the block diagram. It constitutes a definition of feedback control.

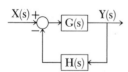

Figure 1.5 Closed loop—canonical form. (From B. G. Lipták (ed.) *Instrument Engineers' Handbook* (Vol. II). Philadelphia: Chilton, 1970.)

Feedback control is that technique which maintains a selected variable in a process, by comparing that variable with its desired value and acting on the process in a manner so as to reduce the deviation between that variable and its desired value. In words this describes the meaning of the block diagram. In the block, G is considered the forward element and H the feedback element.

SUMMARY

Biomedical instrumentation is an interdisciplinary study of interdisciplinary subjects. Biological processes fit into the same pattern as systems analysis of mechanical or chemical processes, or of complex political or management systems. Cybernetics ties all these disciplines together by the feedback principle. Physiology, the study of the function of living organisms, finds feedback in the form of homeostasis, the technique which the organism uses to preserve itself in the presence of outside disturbances. The systems analysis of the entire organism can be broken down into analyses of the subsystems, such as respiration, circulation, the nervous system, the digestive system, and the cell and its subsystems (endoplasmic reticulum and mitochondria).

The science of instrumentation establishes the accuracy of a measurement by comparison with a standard, and the precision of a measurement by statistical evaluation of repeated measurements with the same instrument. Primary, secondary, and international standards have been established for the fundamental quantities of mass, length, and time, and for derived quantities such as temperature, current, voltage, and resistance. Transducers are used to convert a physiologic measurement to an electronic or mechanical signal which can be studied, recorded, or controlled. Displacement, force, and temperature transducers are described, and the field of analysis instrumentation is introduced.

One of the reasons for the use of instrumentation is to provide numbers which can be used in mathematical models. The flow diagram is a basic tool of the model builder. Each block on the flow diagram represents the transfer function of a specific element in the system. Because these elements are considered linear (they can be manipulated without interaction), the principle of superposition is applied, and a model can be built by combining the elements in the same pattern as is found in the actual system. Testing the model now consists of performing experiments on the model and comparing the results with those obtained from the instrumentation attached to the real system.

EXERCISES

1. Draw the block diagram of a hot-water heater. The desired temperature of the water is compared with the measured temperature, and action is taken to turn on the gas and heat the water when the temperature drops.

2. Draw the block diagram of the control of the temperature of the human body (not fever). When the body becomes too hot, perspiration is increased

to reduce the temperature. The desired temperature is located in the hypothalamus, the area of the brain that controls the temperature recovery functions of the body.

3. Draw a block diagram of a man driving a car along the highway. Consider only his attempt to maintain the car at a fixed position on the highway. His brain compares his actual position with his desired position and sends signals to his muscles to turn the steering wheel properly. An additional transfer function, G_2, connects the motion of the steering wheel with the actual position of the car on the road.

4. Draw a block diagram of the breathing control mechanism. According to the Hering-Breuer reflex, there are receptors in the lungs sensitive to stretch. Hence, on inspiration the lungs expand until these receptors advise the inspiratory control center. They inhibit inspiration and start the expiration process when the stretch set point is reached.

General Literature Cited and References

Beckwith, T. G., and Buck, N. L. Mechanical Measurements. Reading, Mass.: Addison-Wesley, 1969.

Considine, D. M. Process Instruments and Controls Handbook. New York: McGraw-Hill, 1957.

Crichton, M. Five Patients. New York: Knopf, 1970.

Del Toro, V. Principles of Electrical Engineering. Englewood Cliffs: Prentice-Hall, 1965.

Dransfield, P. Engineering Systems and Automatic Control. Englewood Cliffs: Prentice-Hall, 1968.

Guyton, A. C. Textbook of Medical Physiology. 3d ed., Philadelphia: Saunders, 1966.

Lion, K. S. Instrumentation is Scientific Research. New York: McGraw-Hill, 1959.

Minnar, E. J. (editor) ISA Transducer Compendium. New York: Plenum, 1963.

Ruch, T. C., and Patton, H. D. Physiology and Biophysics (19th ed.). Philadelphia: Saunders, 1965.

Chapter 2

The Electronics
of Instrumentation

BIOMEDICAL INSTRUMENTATION is primarily electronic. A sensor detects the variable and converts it by means of an attached transducer to an electronic signal. An appropriate electrical bridge improves the signal, and an amplifier increases its power so that it can sound an alarm or operate a pointer, a scanning dot on an oscilloscope, or a control device. Moreover, cybernetics has provided tools for the recognition of signals in noisy electronic systems—and biological systems are often, if not always, accompanied by artifacts and interfering signals.

The analysis of electrical systems follows the procedure for the analysis of any dynamic system. First we must identify the elements of the system, the energy sources and energy sinks, and the equations of dissipation for each component. The transfer function thus provided for each block may now be combined into larger systems the function of which, for our purposes, will be the obtaining of information from biological sources, its conversion to useful signals, and the use and interpretation of those signals.

The elements of electronic systems are what the electrical engineer terms *lumped parameters*. This process of lumping is typical for system analysis, and we shall examine it in some detail. The three elements of electrical systems are resistance, inductance, and capacitance. We shall soon go into greater detail concerning the nature of these parameters, but for now, assuming that each one has been defined, let us note the abstraction performed when we apply the "lumped parameter" technique.

One form of a resistance is a wound wire. The wire itself has a uniform resistance per unit length, since it is wound into a coil; it has some inductance, and between the coiled wires there is some capacitance. Yet, when we draw the resistor in a circuit, we show it only as a resistance. We ignore the inductance and the capacitance; we assume that all the resistance in the circuit is concentrated at one point. The distributed parameter has been abstracted into a lumped parameter to simplify the analysis.

ELEMENTS OF ELECTRICAL CIRCUITS

The elements of electrical circuits can be divided into *active elements* and *passive elements*. The active elements are the energy sources, such as the voltage and current sources. The passive elements are the resistors, capacitors, inductors, and energy sinks. What about the tubes and transistors? They have both active and passive parts. The tube has resistance between its plate and its cathode; it also has capacitance. The tube is connected to a voltage source, but the current that flows through the tube is more than that supplied by the source. Inside the tube there is a *dependent active source* which generates a voltage that is some multiple of the signal input (the amplification factor of the tube). Thus, we can represent a tube by an *equivalent circuit* which contains nothing but active and passive elements, if we show that one of the active elements is a dependent active element. A similar analysis applies to the transistor.

RESISTANCE

Resistance is best explained by analogy to a flow system. When water is pumped through a pipe, there is resistance to the flow, which can be measured as the difference in pressure between the ends of the pipe. Similarly, when electrical current is made to flow through a copper wire, there is a difference in voltage between the ends of the wire (Figure 2.1). Whereas the flow of the water is a function of the square root of the pressure drop,

$$q = CA \sqrt{\frac{2g(P_1 - P_2)}{\rho}}$$

the electrical parameters turn out to be linear,

$$I = (V_1 - V_2)/R$$

Ohm's law equates $V_1 - V_2 = E$, where E is the electromotive force (e.m.f.) represented by the difference in potential $V_1 - V_2$, and we have

$$I = E/R$$

or the potential drop

$$E = IR$$

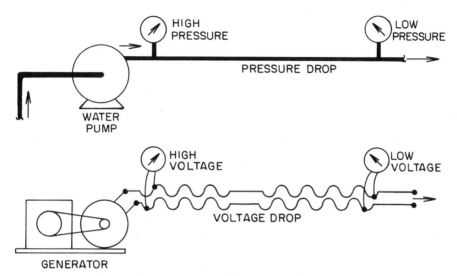

Figure 2.1   Analogy between current flow and water flow.

The power required for this effort is given in volt-amperes or watts. If we had a direct current, the power would be the direct product of a constant voltage and a constant current,

$$P = IE = IIR = I^2R$$

In an alternating current circuit, however, I and E are vectors and may be out of phase with each other. In this case the power

$$P = IE \ (\cos \phi)$$

where ϕ is the power factor, the angle between the current and the voltage. The power is still I^2R, but the current to be used is the effective current I_{eff}. Hence,

$$P_{ac} = I^2_{eff}R$$

Resistance then is the measure of the power dissipation in a circuit, as well as being the measure of the opposition of a piece of material to the flow of current. Each circuit has an equivalent resistance which appears across the input to the system. This can be the physical resistance of the wire in the circuit or it can be based on the power dissipation of the circuit. *Ohmic* resistance is used as a measure of the first condition; *input* resistance may be used as a definition of the second.

The input resistance of a component can be determined by measuring the instantaneous voltage and current entering that device. For example, in Figure 2.2 resistance is the slope of the e-i curve at any point, i.e.,

$$R = de/di$$

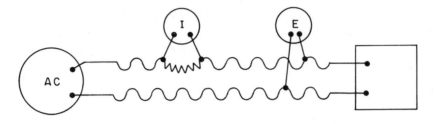

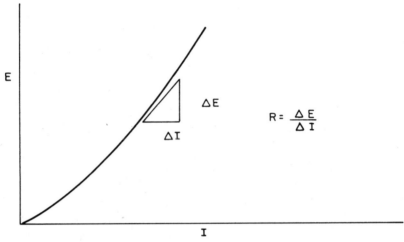

Figure 2.2 Input resistance measurement.

In words, resistance is the ratio of the potential change to the change in current produced.

INDUCTANCE

In 1831 Faraday determined that a voltage is induced in a coil of wire every time the current changes, in particular, on opening and closing the circuit. When alternating current flows through a wire the current is always changing. If the wire is properly coiled, the magnetic field generated will cut across the wires as the field moves in and out with the alternation of the current. The moving magnetic field will generate a voltage in the coil of wire. The inductance of the coil is its tendency to self-induction, L in the equation

$$e = L\ di/dt$$

If more than one coil is used, it is possible to use that coil to induce a voltage in a second coil (as in a transformer). This is called mutual induction, and the inductance M is used to explain this condition.

Although the electrical engineer tends to represent L and M by the same symbol (L), we shall keep them separate in order to explain a biomedical phenomenon that appears in *impedance plethysmography*.

CAPACITANCE

Capacitance is the ability of a circuit to store energy in the electrical field. The electrical field stored on two parallel plates would be affected by 1) the area of the plates; 2) the distance between the plates; 3) the material between the plates (air, oil, insulation); and 4) the potential energy between the plates. The first three criteria are functions of the geometry and physical nature of the system, and not of the electrical energy. We can say then that

$$Q = CE$$

where Q = quantity of electricity stored, in coulombs
$\quad\quad$ E = the electrical potential
$\quad\quad$ C = the capacitance, a function of the physical construction of the device.

If e and i are changing, the quantity $q = \int idt$

and

$$\frac{dq}{dt} = C\,\frac{de}{dt} = i$$

or

$$e = \frac{1}{C}\int idt$$

As the current flows, a potential is stored in the capacitor in the form of electrical energy. We might also say that C = dq/de, the change in quantity stored per unit change in potential.

IMPEDANCE

When the input to a circuit is alternating current (AC) instead of direct current (DC), i.e., $V_{in} = V_{sin\ wt}$, the output will be sinusoidal but different in phase and amplitude if there is capacitance or inductance present, or both. A very interesting relationship

$$e^{jw} = \cos w + j \sin w$$

can be observed by looking up the series values for e^u, cos w, and sin w:

$$\cos w = 1 - \frac{w^2}{2 \cdot 1} + \frac{w^4}{4 \cdot 3 \cdot 2 \cdot 1} - \cdots$$

$$\sin w = w - \frac{w^3}{3 \cdot 2 \cdot 1} + \frac{w^5}{5 \cdot 4 \cdot 3 \cdot 2 \cdot 1} - \cdots$$

$$e^u = 1 + u + \frac{u^2}{2 \cdot 1} + \frac{u^3}{3 \cdot 2 \cdot 1} + \frac{u^4}{4 \cdot 3 \cdot 2 \cdot 1} + \frac{u^5}{5 \cdot 4 \cdot 3 \cdot 2 \cdot 1}$$

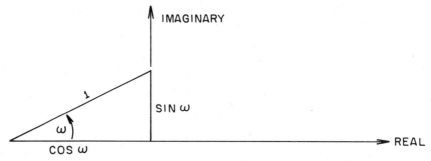

Figure 2.3 Relationship between real and imaginary parts of a function.

This algebraic relationship also has a very interesting geometrical relationship (Fig. 2.3).

If w is the angle between the real and imaginary components of a function, then the vector 1 is the vector sum of cos w + j sin w. The magnitude of this vector is the square root of the sum of the squares of the components:

$$1 = \sin^2 w + \cos^2 w$$

and the angle w

$$w = \tan^{-1} \frac{\text{real part}}{\text{imaginary part}} = \tan^{-1} \frac{\sin w}{\cos w} = \tan^{-1}(\tan w) = w$$

This relationship makes it possible for us to use vectors to represent the input and output to an AC circuit and to analyze circuits by applying circuit laws to the components of vectors.

Impedance—Case 1

If we start with a pure resistance as shown in Figure 2.4, for the DC source,

$$V = IR$$

For the AC source,

$$v = iR$$

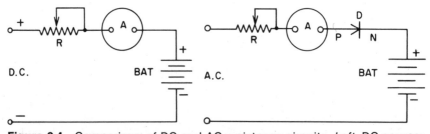

Figure 2.4 Comparison of DC and AC resistance circuits. *Left,* DC source; *Right,* AC source. (From C. R. Cantowine *Battery Chargers and Testers.* Philadelphia: Chilton, 1971.)

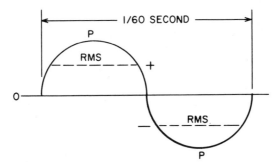

Figure 2.5 Current and voltage in AC circuit (sinusoidal plot). (From C. R. Cantowine *Battery Chargers and Testers*. Philadelphia: Chilton, 1971.)

But

$$v = V \sin wt$$

and since R is not a function of w,

$$i = \frac{V}{R} \sin wt$$

If v is the input and i is the output, the output would be in phase with the input but would be reduced in magnitude by division by R. If the magnitude of i is represented by /i/

$$/i/ = /v/ \cdot \frac{1}{R}$$

and if the angle of i is represented by $\angle i$

$$\angle i = \angle v = 0 = w$$

This checks in exponential notation:

$$e^{jw} = \cos w + j \sin w$$
$$w = 0 \qquad e^0 = 1 = \cos 0 + j \sin 0$$

Impedance—Case 2

When there is inductance or capacitance, or both in a circuit, we use the concept of impedance represented by the vector Z instead of the scalar R, representing the resistance.

For the AC source with impedance Z,

$$v = iZ$$

where v, i, and Z all have magnitudes and directions, and we obtain the product of i and Z by representing each in its exponential form:

$$i = I \sin wt = Ie^{j\phi i}$$

$$Z = /Z/e^{j\phi z}$$

$$v = Ve^{j\phi v}$$

from which

$$Ve^{j\phi v} = IZ \ (e^{j\phi i} \ e^{j\phi z})$$

$$= IZ \ (e^{j\phi i + j\phi z})$$

The magnitude of the product is obtained by multiplying the magnitudes of the vectors; the angle of the product is obtained by adding the angles of the vectors. This would appear as plots on the time and frequency planes (Fig. 2.6).

With I as the input at angle 0 and Z the impedance at angle ϕ_z, the output V would be at angle ϕ_z and of magnitude equal to the magnitude I × the magnitude of Z.

Impedance — Case 3

For a pure inductor,

$$v = \frac{Ldi}{dt}$$

If

$$i = Ie^{j\phi + jwt}$$

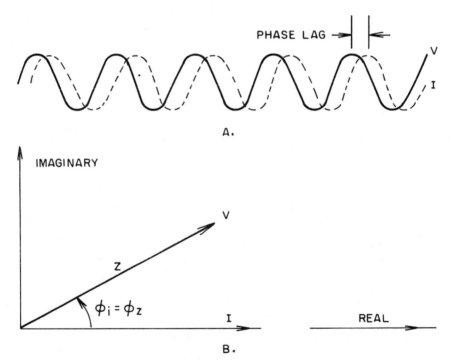

A.

B.

Figure 2.6 Time-frequency plots of V-IZ. *A*, Sinusoidal plot, t plane; *B*, Vector plot, s plane.

and

$$v = Ve^{jwt}$$

$$Ve^{jwt} = LIe^{j\phi}e^{jw} \times j^w$$

from which

$$I = \frac{V}{jwL} \cdot \frac{j}{j} = -j\left(\frac{V}{wL}\right)$$

That is, if V is a sinusoid on the zero axis, I is a sinusoid that lags by an angle the tangent of which = wL and the magnitude of which is $\sqrt{\frac{1+V^2}{(wL)^2}}$.

$$I = V/wL = V/Z$$

we call the L part of Z, X_L, the reactance caused by the inductance. For a pure capacitor, $i = C\frac{dv}{dt}$ and if $v = V \sin wt = Ve^{jwt}$, then $\frac{dv}{dt} = jwVe^{jwt}$

$$i = Ie^{j(wt+\phi)}$$

$$Ie^{j(wt+\phi)} = C(jw)e^{jwt}V$$

$$i = Ie^{j\phi} = j(Cw)V,$$

and if $i = v/Z$, then $X_c = 1/wC$ where X_c is the capacitative reactance in ohms.

Hence in general the impedance $Z = R + j\left(wL - \frac{1}{wc}\right)$ as a vector with magnitude $/Z/ = \sqrt{R^2 + \left(\frac{wL-1}{wC}\right)^2}$ at an angle $\phi_z = \tan^{-1}\frac{wL-(1/wC)}{R}$.

The reactances X_L and X_c are functions of the frequency w.

At the resonant frequency the imaginary parts of the impedance are zero, i.e., $wL - 1/wC = 0$

$$wL = 1/wC$$

$$w^2LC = 1$$

$$w_r = 1/\sqrt{LC}$$

The angular frequency w is in units of radians per second. For the resonant frequency in cycles per second (Hz.)

$$f = w/2\pi = \frac{1}{2\pi}\sqrt{LC}$$

At resonance,

$$/Z/ = R, \Theta_z = 0, \text{ and the current } i = v/R$$

ELECTRICAL CIRCUITS

An electrical circuit is a closed path composed of active and passive elements through which current is made to flow. The current or the voltage of the circuit may communicate a signal, or provide some form of power. Our studies will deal mainly with signal communication.

The active element supplies energy to the circuit, the passive element receives the energy and dissipates or stores it in the form of heat, magnetic energy, or electrical energy. The passive elements are the resistor, the inductor, and the capacitor.

Circuits are also used to represent an analogue of other physical systems. In electronic engineering, transistor circuits are represented by resistances and active elements. Because some of the active elements are dependent on other active elements, transistor circuits are often called active circuits.

KIRCHHOFF'S LAW

The rules that organize the solution of circuit problems are called Kirchhoff's laws. They have both a current form and a voltage form. Kirchhoff's current law states that at any intersection (node) of a circuit, the sum of the currents is equal to zero. Kirchhoff's voltage law states that the sum of the voltages around any loop of a circuit is zero.

Kirchhoff's laws make it possible to calculate the effect of connecting resistors in series and in parallel. In the circuit of Figure 2.7 there are four resistors shown in parallel (R_{11}, R_{21}, R_{22}, and R_{23}).

At node 1, $$I = I_{11} + I_{12}$$

At node 2, $$I_{12} = I_{21} + I_{22} + I_{23}$$

From which

$$I = I_{11} + I_{21} + I_{22} + I_{23}$$

There are also four loops passing through V and each of the R's, but in every loop $I = V/R$

$$I_{11} = V/R_{11}$$

$$I_{21} = V/R_{21}$$

$$I_{22} = V/R_{22}$$

$$I_{23} = V/R_{23}$$

Substituting for the I's in the immediately preceding equations,

$$\frac{V}{R} = \frac{V}{R_{11}} + \frac{V}{R_{21}} + \frac{V}{R_{22}} + \frac{V}{R_{23}}$$

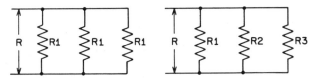

Figure 2.7 Circuit with resistors in parallel. (From C. R. Cantowine *Battery Chargers and Testers.* Philadelphia: Chilton, 1971.)

where R is the equivalent resistance of the entire circuit. Canceling the common V's,

$$\frac{1}{R} = \frac{1}{R_{11}} + \frac{1}{R_{21}} + \frac{1}{R_{22}} + \frac{1}{R_{23}}$$

we arrive at the rule that resistances in parallel add as their reciprocal.

If we note that conductance $(G) = 1/R$, we find that overall conductance

$$G = G_{11} + G_{21} + G_{22} + G_{23}$$

Therefore, conductances in parallel add directly.

In the circuit of Figure 2.8, applying Kirchhoff's laws, the voltage law can be represented as $V = IR_1 + IR_2 + IR_3$.

To obtain equivalent resistance, note that

$$V = IR$$

and

$$IR = IR_1 + IR_2 + IR_3$$

Dividing out the common current

$$R = R_1 + R_2 + R_3,$$

we note that resistances in series do indeed add directly.

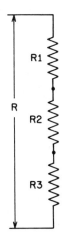

Figure 2.8 Circuit with resistors in series. (From C. R. Cantowine *Battery Chargers and Testers.* Philadelphia: Chilton, 1971.)

CAPACITANCES IN SERIES AND PARALLEL

Applying the same principles to capacitance, we see from Figure 2.9 that

$$I = I_1 + I_2 \quad \text{and} \quad dI = CdE$$

$$dI = dI_1 + dI_2$$

$$CdE = C_1dE + C_2dE$$

$$CdE = (C_1 + C_2)dE$$

When $C = C_1 + C_2$, capacitances in parallel add. By a similar analysis of Figure 2.10 we can see that

$$\frac{1}{C} = \frac{1}{C_1} + \frac{1}{C_2}$$

Therefore, capacitances in series add as their reciprocal.

In the analysis of an R-L-C circuit (Fig. 2.11), the voltage drop across the resistor

$$e_1 = IR,$$

and across the inductor

$$e_2 = L \, di/dt,$$

and across the capacitor

$$e_3 = \frac{1}{C} \int idt.$$

The voltage law around the loop

$$e = e_1 + e_2 + e_3$$

$$e = iR + L \frac{di}{dt} + \frac{1}{C} \int idt$$

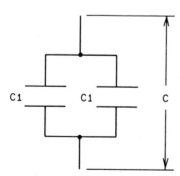

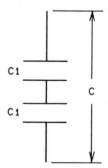

Figure 2.9 Circuit with capacitors in parallel. (From C. R. Cantowine *Battery Chargers and Testers.* Philadelphia: Chilton, 1971.)

Figure 2.10 Circuit with capacitors in series. (From C. R. Cantowine *Battery Chargers and Testers.* Philadelphia: Chilton, 1971.)

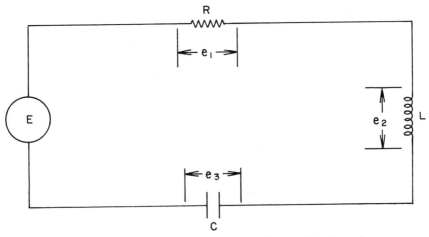

Figure 2.11   Circuit with resistor, inductor and capacitor in series.

ACTIVE CIRCUIT ELEMENTS

VACUUM TUBES

The electron tube is not yet obsolete in biomedical instrumentation. There are still some tasks that only tubes can perform, and until the cathode follower and the high impedance grid have found a replacement, the study of tube theory is still needed. It also helps, in understanding solid-state operations, to start with the study of the electron tube.

The two basic principles required to understand electron behavior in high vacuum involve 1) how electrons are emitted, and 2) how electron emission is controlled. A study of the diode introduces these subjects.

Vacuum Diode

In the diode, thermal energy supplied by the heater causes electrons to leave the metal of the cathode. The positive charge imparted to the plate by the power supply causes the electrons to be conducted to the plate. Besides thermionic emission, light and radioactivity can cause emission of electrons. Special tubes which utilize this principle will be discussed in Chapter 5.

With thermal energy as a source, the number of electrons emitted can be calculated from the equation

$$I_{th} = SA_0 T^2 e^{-E_W/E_T}$$

where S = cathode emitter surface in square meters
   A_0 = a constant characteristic of the material of the cathode
   T = absolute temperature, °K

E_W = work function, in electron-volts
E_T = T/11; 600 is the electron-volt equivalent of temperature T
e = base of natural logarithm

The actual current collected at the plate is a function of the geometry of the tube and the potential at the plate E_b:

$$I_b = KE_b^{3/2}$$

which when plotted produces the operating curve of the diode (Fig. 2.12).

Current flow is proportional to the 3/2 power of plate voltage, but it is restricted by I_{th}, the maximum thermal emission. If more electrons are produced by thermal emission than can be received at the plate, a space charge forms from the excess electrons, and some are repelled back to the cathode.

Vacuum Triode

If a grid is placed between the cathode and plate, the equation for the plate current becomes

$$I_b = K(uE_c + E_b)^n$$

where E_c = grid voltage
u = weighting factor due to close proximity of grid
n ≅ 3/2
K = geometric factor

If a series of curves are plotted based on E_c as a parameter, the characteristic curve is the same for $E_c = 0$ as for the diode. But when, for example, $E_c = -1$ volt, and u = 20, the characteristic curve is shifted to the right until E_b exceeds uE_c, i.e., 20 volts.

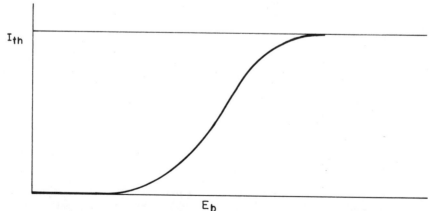

Figure 2.12 Characteristic curve of the diode.

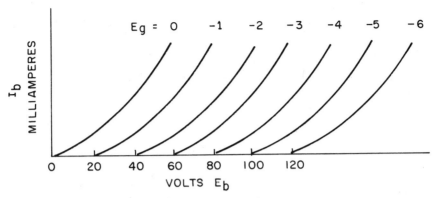

Figure 2.13 Characteristic curve of the triode.

THE SEMICONDUCTOR

The semiconductor gives us the same kind of control over signals that we can obtain with tubes, without the requirement of a heated filament. Instead of transmission of electrons through a vacuum, the semiconductor functions by displacing electrons and holes by diffusion through the crystalline structure of a metal.

A pure tetravalent element such as germanium or selenium is not a conductor. Every electron in the outer shell is bound to the crystalline structure. However, if traces of a pentavalent impurity such as arsenic are added to a pure germanium crystal, the extra valence electron of the arsenic cannot fit into the structure and consequently furnishes a free electron which will diffuse through the crystal under the impetus of a driving force (voltage). The arsenic is termed a *donor* and produces an N-type semiconductor.

On the other hand, when a trivalent atom (indium or gallium, for example) is added to the crystal, one of the positions in the binding lattice is missing, and a vacancy is formed into which an electron can jump from another position in the crystal, leaving a vacancy in *its* place. Thus we have the diffusion of holes in a P-type semiconductor which is doped by an acceptor impurity.

THE P-N JUNCTION

The P-N junction is formed by filling the interstices of a single crystal of germanium while it is being formed, with acceptor atoms in one part of the crystal and donor atoms in another part. The P-N junction will look like Figure 2.14, with holes in the P portion and excess electrons in the N portion.

If electrons from the N side try to diffuse into the P side, they leave positive charges behind them which tend to pull them back. Instead of transmission of electrons through a vacuum, the electrons diffuse through the crystalline structure of a semiconductor, causing an ap-

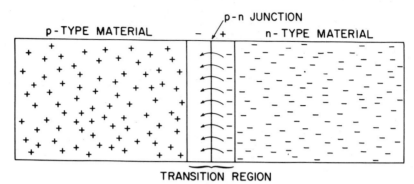

Figure 2.14 P-N junction of a semiconductor. (From J. Berens, and S. Berens *Understanding and Troubleshooting Solid-State Electronic Equipment.* Philadelphia: Chilton, 1969.)

parent displacement of the charges or lack of charges (holes) in the crystal. This potential energy barrier is symbolized by V_0, and is similar to the work function E_W of metals.

If now we close the switch (Fig. 2.15), imposing a potential on the barrier from the battery, with the positive connected to the P material and the negative to the N, the forward bias V will decrease the potential energy barrier from V_0 to $V_0 - V$. For as a hole moves across the junction, another hole is supplied by the battery to maintain electroneutrality, and as an electron moves out of the N region the battery supplies another electron to maintain neutrality in that region. As these electrons and holes move through the junction, a diffusion current is produced which will not be an ohmic current but will have an exponential effect. The total diffusion current is the sum of the current due to holes in the N region and that due to electrons in the P region.

$I = I_{PN} + I_{NP}$ where I_{PN} = exponential $(V/E_T) = e^{V/E_T}$.

The P-N junction diode diffusion current is exponentially related to the forward bias voltage and produces the volt-ampere characteristic shown in Figure 2.16.

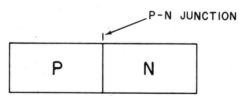

Figure 2.15 Attaching battery to P-N junction. (From B. G. Lipták (ed.) *Instrument Engineers' Handbook* (Vol. II). Philadelphia: Chilton, 1970.)

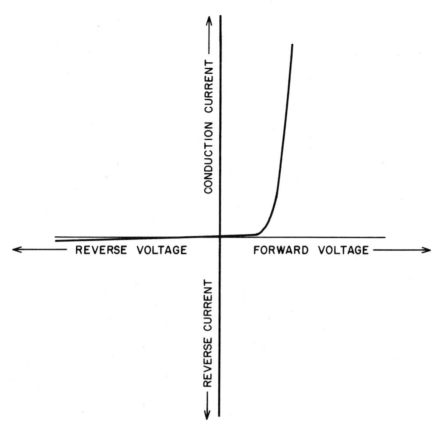

Figure 2.16 Diffusion current of a P-N junction. (From B. G. Lipták (ed.) *Instrument Engineers' Handbook* (Vol. II). Philadelphia: Chilton, 1970.)

THE ZENER DIODE

When reverse bias is applied, the field tries to move holes and electrons from regions in which they are scarce to regions in which they are plentiful. The reverse saturation current is very small as long as V is less than V_0. When a large negative voltage is applied, all the covalent bonds are disrupted and ohmic current flow occurs. In the Zener diode, back voltage between V and V_z produces a constant current I_0, which when passed through a dropping resistor is used to produce a constant voltage (I_0R). The Zener diode is used to replace the battery or standard cell in many instruments as a constant DC reference voltage.

JUNCTION TRANSISTOR

The junction transistor consists of two diode junctions generated on the same semiconductor crystal. The regions may be formed in the area N-P-N or in the order P-N-P, thus forming the two types of transistors illustrated in Figure 2.17.

Analysis of the transistor proceeds as an extension of analysis of the diodes. Assume that all three electrodes of the N-P-N are at ground potential equivalent to two diodes each short circuited. A very small current flows through the external circuit from P-type to N-type. The emitter is now biased negatively and the collector positively as in Figure 2.18. The junction between the emitter and the base will be biased positively, resulting in appreciable current flow, electron current from e to b, and hole current from b to e. The junction between base and collector, biased negatively, would carry a very small current as a diode. A field, however, would be built up in the region, which would attract most of the negatively charged electrons from the

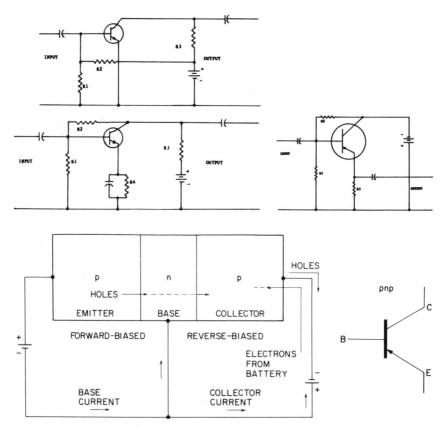

Figure 2.17 Junction transistors and symbols. *A*, NPN transistor; *B*, Emitter-follower circuit. (Part A and B from L. G. Sands *Electronics Handbook for the Electrician*. Philadelphia: Chilton, 1968.) *C*, PNP transistor and short-hand symbol. (From J. Berens and S. Berens *Understanding and Troubleshooting Solid-State Electronic Equipment*. Philadelphia: Chilton, 1969.)

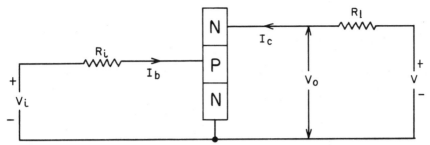

Figure 2.18 Analysis of the transistors. (From B. G. Lipták (ed.) *Instrument Engineers' Handbook* (Vol. II). Philadelphia: Chilton, 1970.)

emitter junction entering the base. A large portion of the emitter current, approximately $\dfrac{i_e a_n}{(a_p + a_n)}$ would appear as the collector current i_c.

If now a voltage signal is applied to the base in a direction to increase i_e, an increase would result in i_c. The transistor can be conceived as a device whose current-carrying capacity is controlled by a relatively small signal at the base.

SIGNAL AMPLIFICATION

Some form of amplification is usually required for each type of biomedical instrumentation system. The vacuum tube triode provides the simplest form of signal amplification. The design of the triode amplifier can be performed graphically on the tube performance chart or can be done analytically, using the equivalent circuit for the vacuum triode. Similarly, the transistor amplifier can be designed either graphically or by use of its equivalent linear circuit. The impedance of the amplifier must be matched to the signal source, and the output of the amplifier must be matched to the display unit. The equivalent circuit techniques provide useful tools for impedance matching. The cathode follower is an amplifier whose gain is less than one, but whose high input impedance provides protection against loading a low impedance source. Operational amplifiers have been developed to amplify DC signals without the usual drift that accompanies a DC amplifier.

VACUUM TUBE TRIODE AMPLIFIER

The amplification in a vacuum tube is based on the principle that the flow of electrons from cathode to plate can be controlled by a small change in grid voltage (Fig. 2.19).

If the cathode is considered at ground potential

     e_c = grid voltage with respect to cathode

     e_b = instantaneous plate voltage with respect to cathode

     i_b = instantaneous current through load resistor

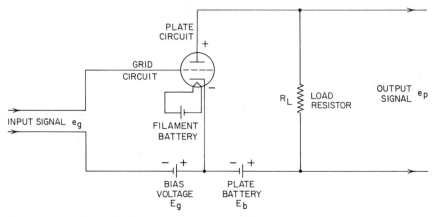

Figure 2.19 Circuit of vacuum tube amplifier.

Applying Kirchhoff's law to the output circuit,

1. $$E_b = e_b + i_b R_L$$

from which we can derive the plate current,

2. $$i_b = \frac{E_b}{R_L} - \frac{1}{R_L} e_b$$

From the tube characteristic curve we have

3. $$i_b = K(u e_c + e_b)^n$$

Since n is not equal to 1, the algebraic solution of these equations is not convenient. The solution is usually performed graphically on the plate characteristic curve (Fig. 2.20).

The triode characteristic curves are reproduced in Figure 2.20 from

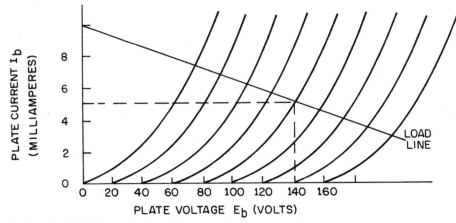

Figure 2.20 Graphical solution of vacuum tube circuit.

Figure 2.13, a graphical reproduction of equation 3. The plot of equation 2 on the same graph produces solutions for comparable values of i_b and e_b for this tube. Thus, when $i_b = 0$, $e_b = 400$ v.; and when $e_b = 0$, $i_b = 8$ ma. Locating these two points on the graph allows for the plot of the load-line.

Applying Kirchhoff's law to the input grid circuit

4.
$$e_c = -E_c + e_g$$

where e_g = grid voltage from an external signal if $E_c = 4$ v., $e_c = -4$ v. when no signal enters.

This is the quiescent operating point, located on the −4 v. line, where the load-line crosses. At this point one can locate the quiescent voltage = 140 v. at a plate current of 4.8 ma. Now if a sinusoidal signal enters

5.
$$e_g = 4 \sin wt$$

6.
$$e_c = -E_c + e_g = -4 + 4 \sin wt$$

Since the sine may vary from 0 to 1 to −1, e_c will vary from −8 to 0, and e_b will vary from 60 v. to 180 v. The amplification factor will be $180 − 60/0 − (−8) = 15$.

EQUIVALENT CIRCUITS OF VACUUM TRIODE

Another method of analysis of the vacuum tube, which will later be applied to transistor circuits, is the equivalent circuit analysis. From the mathematical equations of the vacuum tube one may note the effect of changes in input signal on changes in output signal. A model based on the perturbation of signal about the quiescent operating point considers only the AC character of input and output. It is an AC model of the vacuum triode.

The equivalent model is obtained by replacing the effect of changes of grid voltage on current flow through the tube by a dependent active source. As the source in the grid circuit changes by e_g, the source in the plate circuit changes by ue_g, where u is the amplification factor of the tube.

TRANSISTOR AMPLIFIER

By parallel development we can derive the graphical technique and equivalent circuit analysis for a transistor amplifier. The load curve will make possible the graphical solution of a transistor amplifier as was done for the vacuum tube on Figure 2.20. The equivalent circuit of the transistor amplifier would have current sources instead of voltage sources because the transistor acts as a current amplifier rather than as a voltage amplifier. The transistor can be conveniently represented by a little black box with four terminals (Fig. 2.21).

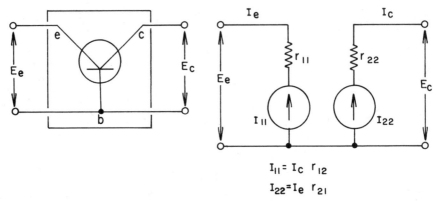

$$I_{11} = I_c \ r_{12}$$
$$I_{22} = I_e \ r_{21}$$

Figure 2.21   Equivalent circuit of transistor amplifier.

In the equivalent circuit shown, the r's represent partial derivatives, i.e.,

$$r_{11} = \frac{\delta e_{be}}{\delta i_e} \qquad r_{12} = \frac{\delta e_{be}}{\delta i_c}$$

$$r_{21} = \frac{\delta e_{bc}}{\delta i_e} \qquad r_{22} = \frac{\delta e_{bc}}{\delta i_c}$$

be refers to subscript 11
bc refers to subscript 12
i_e refers to subscript 21
i_c refers to subscript 22

IMPEDANCE MATCHING

One of the most chronic problems in the use of amplifiers in measuring circuits involves impedance matching. By definition a matched impedance transmits the maximum signal, whereas the unmatched impedance produces loss. A modified version of the equivalent circuit for both transistor and tube provides a tool for the evaluation of the degree of mismatch in the impedance of amplifier versus transducer on one hand, or final display element on the other. An equivalent circuit for an amplifier operating at moderate frequencies (which means in the frequency range for which it was designed) is shown in Figure 2.22.

By way of explanation of this circuit, all input resistances in the amplifier have been replaced by one equivalent resistance R_{in}, and all output resistances by one equivalent resistance R_{out}. All amplifying properties have been replaced by the one voltage amplifier which produces an active output voltage, A × the input voltage, across the output resistance. This simplification can be readily performed by repeated application of Kirchhoff's laws to the input and output networks.

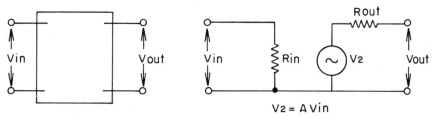

Figure 2.22 Equivalent circuit for evaluating impedance match.

Now, when a signal is brought to the amplifier, we shall represent it by a voltage source and a resistance. The output of the amplifier is connected across a load, represented by a resistance. The essential feature of impedance match now consists in matching these resistances respectively with the input and output resistance of the equivalent circuit. That is, for optimum impedance match, which would provide optimum transmission of signal, R_1 should equal R_{in}, and R_2 should equal R_{out}. If these values are substantially unequal, an impedance matching device should be installed between the input device and the amplifier, or between the output device and the amplifier, or both. Such a device could be a transformer with input resistance R_1, and output resistance, R_{in}. A simple amplifier circuit with these input and output impedances could also be used. The selection of the proper circuit depends on the frequency response required. Transformers tend to attenuate high frequencies, whereas a simple triode amplifier does not.

THE CATHODE FOLLOWER

The cathode follower is a device to aid impedance matching. It has a very high input impedance and a very low output impedance. Connection of a high impedance to a low impedance source will not disturb the source. Hence, the cathode follower can be connected to most transducers without affecting the dynamic frequency response of the signal. On the other side of the circuit, the low output makes it compatible with most output devices. Connected to a meter of low impedance, for example, it will operate most efficiently. Connected to an oscilloscope that normally has a high input impedance, it will not affect the signal unfavorably (although it is not needed in this case). Observe that the input to the amplifier (Fig. 2.23) is a resistor, and thus is a low impedance source; the addition of a cathode follower at this point will produce a high impedance input for delicate, dynamic, low impedance signal sources.

OPERATIONAL AMPLIFIERS

Operational amplifiers were developed originally for the amplification of DC signals in analogue computers. Now in the solid-state, low

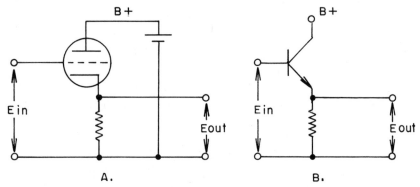

Figure 2.23 Cathode and emitter-follower circuits. *A*, Cathode follower; *B*, Emitter follower.

cost form they are being used increasingly as amplifiers in measuring systems.

A DC amplifier may be constructed in either of two ways. Both methods have been used on operational amplifiers. The first method eliminates all capacitors from interstage coupling and depends on increased stability of power supply and tube (or transistor) to prevent drift. The second method uses a chopper or vibrator to convert the DC signal to an AC type signal, amplifies in the AC mode, and demodulates the signal back to DC after amplification.

The low drift DC amplifier has been constructed with a large load resistance on an input triode. This lowers the load-line shown in Figure 2.20 to where it is nearly horizontal, providing a constant plate current, independent of drift in the emission characteristics. A cathode follower is then used to transfer the signal with maximum stability and with high amplification. Additional amplification again uses a cathode follower output stage for matching to a low impedance display unit.

The chopper-stabilized amplifier may utilize either a mechanical or an electronic chopper. On the mechanical chopper the input switch moves between two contacts, periodically reversing the signal across the input transformer. A standard AC amplifier is used to intensify the signal, and the output signal is demodulated back to DC by a chopper synchronized with the input chopper. The electronic chopper operates in a similar manner, using the DC signal to modulate an oscillator signal. The peak value of the oscillating frequency is proportional to the DC signal.

DISPLAY AND RECORDING EQUIPMENT

No matter how ingenious the measurement technique employed, and how carefully the transducer and amplifier are designed, if the pen runs out of ink there will be no record of the test. Especially in biomedical measurements the ability to record data properly as they occur is essential to the success of the experiment. Early biomedical patient monitors were unpopular because they used reams of chart paper and required constant attention to inking and maintenance of the chart. It was only with the advent of the cathode tube display and the digital readout that biomedical accessories became popular in the hospital.

THE D'ARSONVAL METER

Paradoxically, our measurement system usually starts and ends with a displacement. Most variables are converted to displacements, after which they are transduced into electrical signals which we amplify and transmit to some remote point where we again convert the signal back to a displacement, a pointer moving on the scale of a meter.

The heart of most meters is the D'Arsonval movement, a light coil moving in a cylindrical space between the poles of a magnet. The current flowing through the coil induces a magnetic field which bucks the field from the magnet to move the coil. A spring, or the tension on the coil itself, resists this motion with a torque proportional to the angle of rotation. When the resisting force equals the magnetic force, the needle stops moving and a reading is obtained. The essence of the D'Arsonval movement is that it is sensitive only to direct current.

Meters, however, are used for measurement of voltage as well as current, for AC as well as DC measurement. The input circuit to the meter determines its sensitivity. For measurement of DC flow, the meter is placed directly in the line so that the current through the line flows through the meter. For measurement of voltage, Ohm's law is used. The voltage is made to drop across a resistance and the equivalent current passes through the meter (Fig. 2.24). The resistance is connected across the line, and the voltmeter connected across the resistance.

For measurement of AC the signal is rectified. A half-wave rectifier will supply a pulsating current the average value of which is 31.8% of

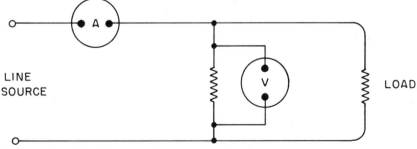

Figure 2.24 The D'Arsonval meter as voltmeter and ammeter.

the peak current. If the meter is properly calibrated for both Ohm's law and this reduction in value, a peak reading voltmeter will be obtained. Usually we desire the root mean square (r.m.s.) value of the voltage. Using the fact that the r.m.s. voltage is equal to 0.707 of the peak value, the meter scale is marked accordingly.

THE VACUUM TUBE VOLTMETER (VTVM)

When a DC voltmeter is attached to a circuit the coil resistance of the meter loads the circuit. A vacuum tube amplifier with a high input impedance will not load the circuit, yet has a response equivalent at least to that of the voltmeter alone. The VTVM may utilize a cathode follower input, may use a difference signal to avoid the effect of tube drift, or may use an additional rectifier stage for use as an AC VTVM. A cathode follower VTVM might look like the one shown in Figure 2.25. To be completely functional it should have the additional components shown in Figure 2.26.

THE VOLT OHMMETER

The volt-ohm-milliammeter (VOM) combines the functions of a voltmeter (Fig. 2.27), an ammeter (milliampere range), and an ohmmeter in one piece of equipment. The voltmeter and the ammeter have been described in this chapter. The ohmmeter consists of an internal battery placed in series with the external resistance and the internal DC ammeter. The instrument is zeroed by shorting the leads and setting the battery so that the meter reads zero. By appropriate resistance networks, the current flowing through the external resistance can be shunted so that only that portion less than the actual range of the meter is passed through the meter. The basic equation of the ohmmeter is $I = E/R$, where I is the current flowing through the meter, E is the fixed voltage source of the battery, and R is the unknown resistance.

CATHODE RAY OSCILLOSCOPE

The oscilloscope (Fig. 2.28) is the answer to an instrument engineer's dream. It has all the features that make for good measurement display. It has a high input impedance so that it will not load the measurement bridge. It has rapid response so that dynamic signals can be displayed. Fast signals like the pulses passing through the nerves may be observed. It has adjustable range from 0.01 v. to 10 v. per division, and adjustable speed from microseconds to 1 second per division. The only problem is that the readout is not permanent; it may be observed, even stored, for a short period of time, but eventually it will fade from the screen.

The cathode ray tube is the heart of the oscilloscope. It has a fluorescent screen upon which electrons record the signal. The mo-

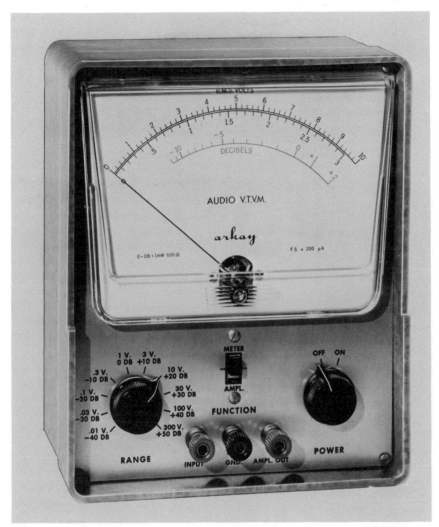

Figure 2.25 Cathode follower VTVM. (From L. G. Sands *Electronics Handbook for the Electrician.* Philadelphia: Chilton, 1968.)

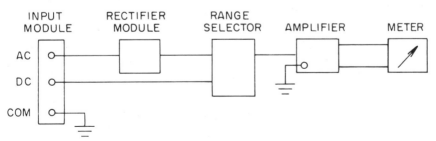

Figure 2.26 Block diagram of functional VTVM.

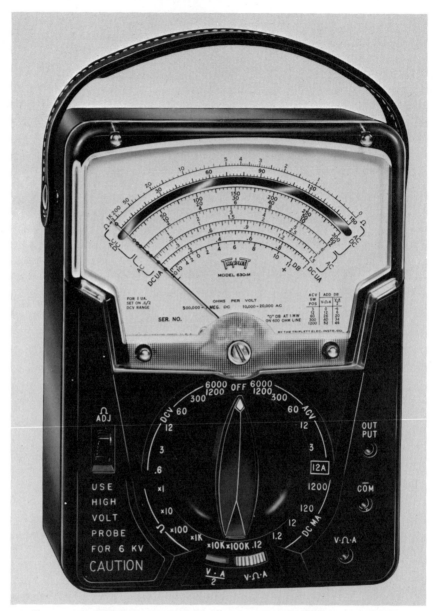

Figure 2.27 Volt-ohm-milliammeter. (From L. G. Sands *Electronics Handbook for the Electrician.* Philadelphia: Chilton, 1968.)

tion of the electrons is controlled by vertical and horizontal deflection plates, the amount of deflection being proportional to the voltage. It is possible to place one signal on the x plate and another on the y plate so as to obtain a plot of x against y. Such a plot is called a Lissajous figure.

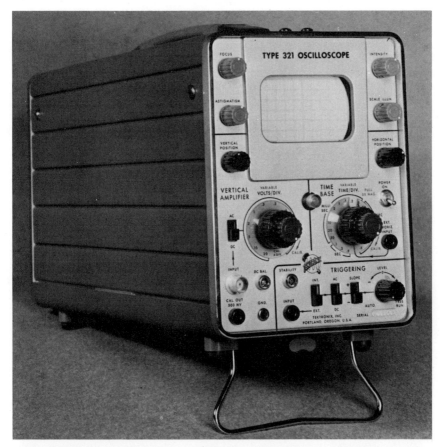

Figure 2.28 Portable, battery-operated oscilloscope. Since it is independent of power lines, it is particularly useful in electronic systems maintenance. (From L. G. Sands *Electronics Handbook for the Electrician.* Philadelphia: Chilton, 1968.)

MODES OF OPERATION OF OSCILLOSCOPE

Normal Mode

In the normal mode of operation, the horizontal amplifier is connected to the sweep generator, and the vertical amplifier displays the signal. Thus a plot of the signal against time is obtained. If the signal is sinusoidal and the horizontal sweep is properly timed so that a single cycle appears on the scope, a pure sine wave will be observed. If the signal is an ECG, if it is regular, and if the rate is predictable, the sweep rate can be adjusted to obtain one, two, or three beats per cycle.

Lissajous Mode

In the Lissajous mode, a second signal is connected to the horizontal amplifier, and the phase relationship between the signals is displayed on the screen. If the signals are in phase, a 45° straight line will appear. If the signals are 90° out of phase, a circle will appear. If the signals are out of phase at any other angle an ellipse will appear, sloping to the right if the angle is between 0° and 90° and to the left if it is between 90° and 180°. At a phase lag of 180° a line at 135° will appear on the screen.

Automatic Mode

In the automatic sweep mode, additional elements will be brought into the picture. It is possible to have the sweep start always at the same position in the vertical signal. Thus, if the signal is a sinusoid the sweep can be started when the sinusoid is at midpoint of the curve (zero voltage) or the curve can be started at any preselected voltage. This operation is a decided advantage when one wants to see a complete ECG cycle, the P-Q-R-S-T wave. (See Chapter 7.) We can set the trigger so that the display starts at the beginning of a cycle rather than in the middle of the R wave.

AUTOMATIC SYNCHRONIZATION

The additional components required for automatic synchronization of an oscilloscope include the Schmitt trigger, differentiator, negative clipper and Miller sweep circuits. The signal going into the vertical deflection plates also enters the Schmitt trigger, where a rectangular pulse is produced, the leading edge of which coincides with the desired position on the y curve. The differentiator converts these wide pulses into sharp impulses (since the derivative goes to infinity at the leading and trailing edge of each step). To remove the second downward impulse a negative clipper is used, leaving only the upward positive peaks. A Miller sweep generator is a stubborn saw-tooth generator. The generator is initiated by the positive pulse, but once started it continues until it has completed its cycle. It therefore generates a traverse across the cathode ray tube, but does not repeat until the complete traverse is made. Thus, if the ECG cycle is one second and the sweep rate across the tube is 0.5 seconds per division, there will be 5 cycles of the ECG for every traverse of the tube (there being 10 divisions in the X direction across the tube.)

RECORDING SYSTEMS

Despite the reams of paper that accumulate when a measurement is made, there is always a desire to record that measurement. Hence, we use mechanical, electrical, or photographic means to convert biomedical information into marks on a chart, or numbers in an automatically printed table, or photographs from an oscilloscope, or magnetic pulses on a tape. And the chart paper, the photographs, and the magnetic tape accumulate.

TYPES OF RECORDERS

1. The direct writing *oscillograph* employs a galvanometer connected to a pen or stylus (Fig. 2.29). The pen inks the paper, or the stylus scratches the wax lines revealing a darker undercoat, or a heated stylus burns marks into the paper. The galvanometer has the same effect on the measurement as the DC meter described in this chapter. It loads down the signal and does not respond to very rapid changes in signal. Commercial oscillographs used for recording physiologic or medical data usually come equipped with preamplifiers, often with cathode follower inputs (emitter followers are the semiconductor version), but in most cases have some high impedance input which does not disturb the signal. Oscillographic recorders are used in the frequency range of 1 to 100 Hz.

2. In *galvanometer light beam recorders,* the light beam is deflected by a mirror attached to the galvanometer, providing no mechanical load and therefore giving higher frequency response. Useful to 1000 Hz, the light beam writes on photosensitive paper, which is developed by the ultraviolet light present in sunlight or fluorescent lamps.

3. *X-Y recorders* contain two servomotors driving the pen in the x

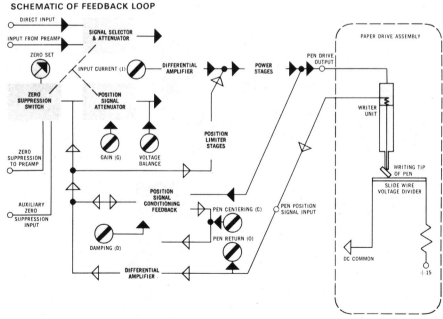

Figure 2.29 Schematic of a direct writing oscillograph. (Courtesy of Beckman Instruments, Inc., Fullerton, California.)

and y direction, respectively. Rapid plotting of any dependent-independent variable combination is possible. The dynamic change in the signal must be slower than that for the oscillograph.

4. *Potentiometric recorders* operate on the self-balancing principle. They cannot operate at speeds higher than ¼-second full scale, and the standard models are much slower. These are the accepted recorders for thermocouples, hot-wire filaments, resistance thermometers, and other millivoltage measurements.

5. In *force balance servorecorders,* a servomotor moves the pen proportionately to the size of the input signal. The balance system matches the input force generated by a current in a coil, with an output force that moves the pen to the proper position on the chart, which compensates for offset due to pen friction on the chart.

6. *Event recorders* have only two positions, on and off. They are used to record the "on time" of events, or the sequence of several operations by many pens on the same chart, each of which has only two positions.

7. *Multiple styli recorders* provide many records on the same chart. They make possible the comparison of many variables with each other, e.g., blood pressure and ECG record on same chart.

8. *Sweep-balance recorders* scan the chart, and a solenoid taps the pen to make a dot when the recorder position matches the input signal—a low-cost but very inaccurate system.

9. *Oscilloscope camera recorders* are cameras that make a permanent record of oscilloscope traces when triggered manually by the researcher or automatically by the system.

10. *Pressure recorders* are pneumatic recorders in which bellows respond to pressure signals to move the pen to the proper position on the chart. Linkages and the spring constant of the bellows provide the calibration and the limitation to dynamic change.

11. *Filled-system (filled-bulb) temperature recorders* place the thermometer directly on the chart. A temperature bulb filled with liquid provides actuation through a capillary for the motion of the pen on the chart.

12. *Special purpose recorders* include the remainder of recording possibilities. For example, the seismograph, built especially for the recording of earth vibrations, contains an arm connected directly to the earth, which moves the pen on the recorder. The kymograph is the physiologist's version of a seismograph, since it contains an arm which can be connected directly to a muscle to record its motion under isotonic and isometric conditions.

The twelve types of recorders can be subdivided into the following five classifications:

1. Moving coil instruments, utilizing a galvanometer motion actuated by a current, to move the pen of the recorder.

2. Self-balancing instruments, which use an electrical or pneumatic

servomotor to position the pen so that the signal generated by the instrument is balanced by the recorder.

3. Electrical bridge instruments with an input conditioning system containing a bridge, and one of the already described modes of operation of the pen.

4. Directly actuated recorders, in which the sensing element is directly connected to the pen. A pressure recorder which feeds the measured pressure into a bellows which moves the pen, is an example.

5. Tape and photographic recorders, including tape recorders which later play back through an oscilloscope, or photographic records which may be later played back in conjunction with moving and still pictures.

DIGITAL DISPLAY

Just as the VTVM is the heart of the analog display, the digital voltmeter (DVM) is the heart of the digital display. The digital voltmeter converts a voltage to a digital signal, usually directly to a display. Since, by proper diligence and application, all the measurements can be converted to voltages, by use of the DVM all the measurements can be displayed digitally. At a nurse's station associated with a bedside monitor of almost any type, a digital display is provided, showing body temperature at 98.6°F (real digits), arterio-venous pressure or systolic and diastolic blood pressure in mm. Hg, and pulse rate in pulsations per minute.

How is a digital display derived from a voltage signal? Two methods are employed. Either 1) we convert the input voltage to another variable, such as frequency or charge, and then use a counter to count the pulses for a given period of time, or 2) we compare the measured voltage with an internally generated voltage, changing the internal voltage until they match, and when they match, display the voltage. The former is the indirect method, the latter the direct method.

In the indirect method, a pulse generator is used to generate a pulse whose width is proportional to the voltage measured. An accurate 1 mega-Hz. (1,000,000 cycles per second) oscillator is connected with the pulse generator to an AND gate. The AND gate conducts only when both signals are active. Hence, it will transmit the 1 mega-Hz. signal for as long as the pulse is on. The pulses from the AND gate are transmitted to a counter which is calibrated in terms of the original voltage. That is, if the original voltage was 100 volts, the pulse would be on until 10,000 pulses were transmitted—a duration of 0.01 second. The counter would count to 10,000, but the display would be shown as 100.00 volts. The decimal point on the counter would appear in the proper position for calibration of the original signal.

In an instrument using the direct method, a reference voltage is stepped through a series of transistor switches which provides a metered potential, which is matched against the input potential by a null detector. When the null detector senses balance, the setting of the switching transistors is displayed on the meter to the appropriate scale.

SUMMARY

Electronics defines the ground rules for instrumentation. All we can use are electrical circuits which contain passive elements (resistors, capacitors, and inductors) and active elements (current and voltage sources). The sources provide the electrical energy to activate the passive elements. The passive elements dissipate the energy or store it in electrical or magnetic fields. Kirchhoff's voltage and current laws are sufficient to analyze most circuits. Even vacuum tubes and transistors can be represented by equivalent circuits analyzable by Kirchhoff's laws.

By virtue of these circuits we can provide vacuum tubes or transistor systems that will amplify the signals, match the impedance of the instruments, and display or record the measurement. The DC meter furnishes a display of output but also places a load on the instrument. The VTVM supplies equally accurate display but does not load the measuring circuit. A cathode ray oscilloscope will provide a display of signals as fast as 1 mega-Hz. Recording systems, however, will capture only 100 Hz. signals; a mirror galvanometer and light pen will capture 1000 Hz. signals. A storage system can hold the signals and return them later for digital display.

EXERCISES

1. For the circuit shown in Figure 1, calculate the current flow and the potential difference across each resistor.

2. For the circuit shown in Figure 2, calculate the current flow through each branch, and the total current flow. Calculate the potential difference across each resistor.

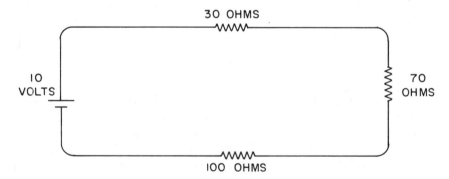

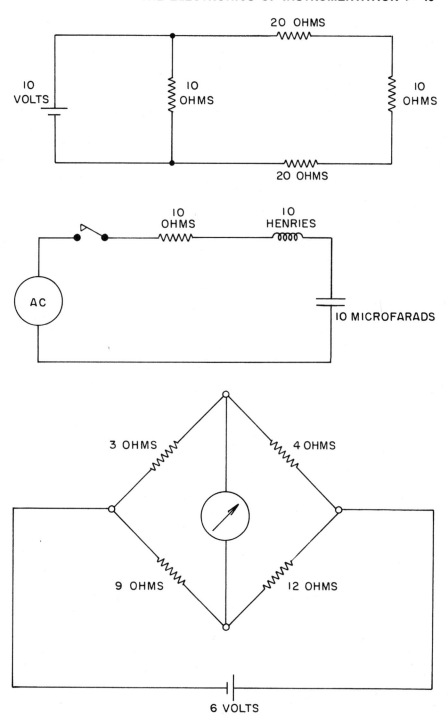

3. The circuit shown in Figure 3 is supplied with 110 v. at 60 Hz. Calculate the initial current flow when the switch is closed, and the steady-state voltage drop across each element.

4. At balance the voltage at point 3 equals that at point 4, in Figure 4. Calculate the ratio of the resistors at balance, the current flow through each branch, and the voltage drop through each resistor.

General Literature Cited and References

Del Toro, V. Principles of Electrical Engineering. Englewood Cliffs: Prentice-Hall, 1965.

Malvino, A. P. Electronic Instrumentation Fundamentals. New York: McGraw-Hill, 1967.

Nilsson, J. W. Introduction to Circuits Instruments and Electronics. New York: Harcourt, Brace & World, 1968.

Shea, R. F. (editor) Amplifier Handbook. New York: McGraw-Hill, 1966.

Weed, H., and Davis, W. L. Fundamentals of Electron Devices and Circuits. Englewood Cliffs: Prentice-Hall, 1959.

Chapter 3

Electrical Transducers

ELECTRICAL SIGNALS are easily amplified, attenuated, filtered, detected, modulated, transmitted, and recorded; but nature has chosen to provide her variables in mechanical, chemical, or physical form. We outwit nature by using transducers to convert measurements of temperature, pressure, flow, volume, pulse rate; chemical properties of blood; respiratory system volume, pressure and flow; body motions; and the stress in isotonic and isometric conditions on bones and muscle to useful electrical signals.

We have reserved the chemical transducers for discussion in Chapters 4 and 5, and are therefore limiting this chapter to the discussion of physical and mechanical measurements.

We shall soon see that a great many of the measurements desired can be converted mechanically to a displacement. Measurement of force, when applied to an elastic element, becomes a displacement. Measurement of temperature with a mercury-in-glass clinical thermometer is the observation of a displacement. We shall find other means to convert temperature to an electrical signal by the use of temperature-sensitive resistors and by thermocouples which generate voltages dependent on the temperature. Pressure measurements can be converted to forces which in turn are displacement measurements. Flow measurements are not readily converted to pressures in the circulatory system, since any obstruction will cause difficulty, and special flow sensors utilizing ultrasound and electromagnetic effects are used. Radiation transducers go directly from the energy source to an electrical signal, because electrical circuits (tubes) are sensitive to radiation.

Having converted our biological signals to electrical signals, we find that they are still wanting. They are not of sufficient magnitude or power to be useful. Hence, we shall propose the use of bridges to modify our signals into useful levels of impedance and size. We shall examine direct current resistance bridges for the various types of DC measurements made. The laboratory bridge balanced by the experimenter will be replaced by the self-balancing bridge, balanced by the servomotor, and eventually by the unbalanced bridge, producing a deflection on a meter. Voltage-sensitive bridges are provided for those transducers that emit voltages from their measuring circuits. Alternating current bridges are provided for impedance balancing of capacitance or inductance signals.

These conversion devices constitute our primary transducers and their signal modifiers, which we shall find used in the biomedical instrumentation described in subsequent chapters.

DISPLACEMENT TRANSDUCERS

Length-measuring devices, from yardsticks to tapes to carpenter's rules, are available in the average novelty store. They measure length by direct comparison, as does the clinical thermometer, which places a scale next to the mercury column for optical comparison. Most instrumental applications, however, require an indirect measurement of displacement which converts that displacement to a useful electrical signal.

Many electrical properties can be modified by displacement. Electrical resistance can be modified by moving a slider across a linear resistance. A pair of coils the magnetic forces of which are linked by a metal core can provide a transformer whose transformation ratio is proportional to the displacement of the core. Or the inductance or reluctance of a magnetic circuit can be modified by displacement. Since the capacitance is a function of the distance between two plates, it can readily be seen that capacitance can be used to measure displacement. There are piezoelectric transducers, which generate an electric potential when squeezed, that can be used to measure displacement.

Mechanical transducers are also useful in measuring displacement. The flapper-nozzle-combination is the heart of the pneumatic control system used in petroleum and chemical plants. But it is not used in biomedical measurements because of the predilection for electronics by biomedical workers.

LINEAR POTENTIOMETER

The linear potentiometer is a device which converts a displacement to a change in resistance. A sliding contact on a resistance coil con-

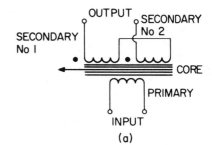

Figure 3.1 Linear potentiometer. (From S. E. Summer *Electronic Sensing Controls.* Philadelphia: Chilton, 1969.)

verts displacement to the variation in resistance of the coil (Fig. 3.1). By connecting a voltage or current source across the coil the measurement can be converted into voltage or current, which may be transmitted to a display meter or used in a computer or other device. The potentiometer is very accurate and very simple to operate. The source and the meter are all that is required to operate the device. Potentiometers are not influenced by vibration or acceleration, but require precision machining. Their resolution is limited to the resistance of a single coil. If 1000 turns are used on a coil, the resolution is $1/1000$ of the measurement or 0.1%. Potentiometers are used for measurements of displacements which occur relatively slowly, for example, less than 1 cycle per second.

DIFFERENTIAL TRANSFORMER

The linearly variable differential transformer (LVDT) provides an AC voltage output proportional to displacement of a core passing through the windings (Fig. 3.2). It is a mutual inductance device using three coils arranged as shown in the figure. The center coil is energized from an external power source by alternating current. The two end coils are used as pickup coils. The magnetic field generated by the center coil is conducted to the end coils by the displacement of the core. At the null position, equal voltages are induced in both coils. Since the coils are wired in opposition, this produces an output of zero volts. Motion in either direction from the null position unbalances the currents induced in the two coils, producing a rapidly linear increasing output. The range, although linear, is very small, providing for a very sensitive measurement in the order of 0.5 mv. per $1/1000$ inch. Laboratory units are available sensitive to 1 microvolt per 1×10^{-6} (one-millionth) inch.

VARIABLE INDUCTANCE TRANSDUCER

A variable inductance transducer element contains one or more inductance coils whose geometry is modified by the displacement being measured. A current flowing through a coil produces a magnetic field. If the current is of the AC type, the magnetic field appears to move

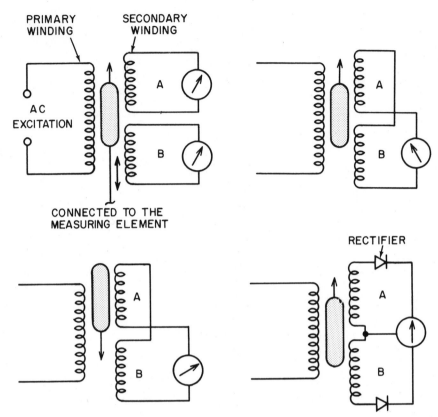

Figure 3.2 Differential transformer. (From B. G. Lipták (ed.) *Instrument Engineers' Handbook* (Vol. II). Philadelphia: Chilton, 1970.)

across the coil with each cycle of current. Motion of a magnetic field induces a voltage in the wire. The inductance of a coil L is the amount of voltage produced by a unit change in the current.

$$E = L \, di/dt$$

When the coil is squeezed by the displacement being measured, L is changed, and if di/dt is maintained constant, the induced voltage E will change proportionally.

Instead of modifying the coil itself, the usual variable inductance transducer modifies the magnetic path provided adjacent to the coil; this is known as modification of the permeability of the flux path. A change in the air gap will produce a change in the meter reading, owing to change in self inductance of the coil. If there were two coils, a change in air gap would effect the permeability of the flux path between the coils, producing an output change proportional to displacement.

VARIABLE RELUCTANCE TRANSDUCER

When a permanent magnet is included in the configuration (Fig. 3.5) the term *variable reluctance* is used instead of variable inductance. The magnetic field of the magnet cuts the wires in the coil, generating an induced voltage only when the reluctance of the magnet is disturbed by the approach of another magnetic material. The displacement of the serrated rack will produce pulses in the readout device, each pulse representing a displacement equal to the width between two teeth (d in Figure 3.3).

CAPACITIVE TRANSDUCER

Capacitive devices provide the highest sensitivity for displacement of the devices already described, but they require more sophisticated electronics for activation and detection. Cylindrical capacitors with a small cylindrical air gap have been used over a large range of displacement measurements. Parallel plate capacitors can measure displacements with a sensitivity of 1×10^{-7} inches.

PIEZOELECTRIC TRANSDUCERS

Some materials possess the property of generating an electrical potential when subjected to mechanical strain. A piezoelectric crystal generates a charge which is nearly proportional to a rapidly applied force. The charge may result from a compression, bending, or shear of the surface of the material caused by a displacement. The charge of the crystal can be measured by a cathode follower (Chapter 2.), emitter follower, or similar high impedance charge amplifier. A large output is produced.

FLAPPER-NOZZLE TRANSDUCER

This device is a common component of pneumatic control systems. By positioning a flapper before a nozzle containing air under pressure,

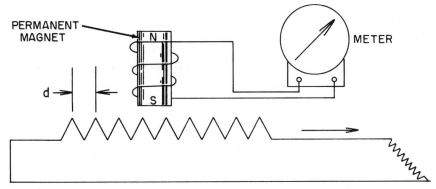

Figure 3.3 Variable reluctance transducer.

with a suitable constriction in the supply line, the output pressure of the configuration will vary with displacement. Sensitivity of 1 inch of water pressure to 0.001 inch displacement is readily obtainable.

FORCE TRANSDUCERS

Force can be measured by observing its ability to compress, bend, or distort an elastic element. The most common elastic element used is the spring. In the spring balance, the forces stretch the spring by an amount proportional to its intensity, moving an attached pointer over a calibrated linear scale. Large static loads are measured with a proving ring, which uses a similar principle. The deflection of the proving ring by the load is measured by an accurate micrometer.

Strain gauge load cells are popularly used for measuring force. The deflection of a member of the load cell produces a strain on the wire of the strain gauge. The stretching of the wire changes its dimensions and hence changes the electrical resistance of the strain gauge, which in turn is measured by a resistance bridge. Since the wire is directly strained, this technique is called an unbonded strain gauge. In a subsequent discussion we shall describe the bonded strain gauge.

The unbonded strain gauge is also used to measure force directly. When the strain is on the wire itself, only small forces can be measured. One family of such gauges has a range of 0.15 ounces to 1000 pounds.

Force transducers are available that produce variable reluctance or motion of a linear differential transformer, or squeeze a piezoelectric crystal, as described in this chapter. The force is applied to a calibrated beam whose distortion by the force can be measured as a displacement.

THE STRAIN GAUGE

Strain is defined by mechanical engineers as $\frac{\Delta L}{L}$, the change in length divided by the original length. The strain gauge is wire whose length is changed when the length of the original sample is changed. The strain gauge is bonded to the sample and feels the strain applied. A strain gauge wire has the property of changing in resistance as it is strained. Stretching a wire increases its length and decreases its cross-sectional area. Since

$$\text{resistance} = k\,\frac{L}{A}$$

where k = specific resistivity
  L = length
  A = area

a general relationship between electrical and mechanical properties may be derived as follows:

$$\text{The cross-sectional area } A = CD^2$$

where C is a constant dependent on the geometry, and D is the diameter. Thus if the section is circular, $C = \pi/4$; if it is square $C = 1$. If the conductor is strained axially

1. $$R = kL/A$$

To find dR/R, the fractional change in R with respect to R we differentiate,

2. $$dR = \frac{A(kdL + Ldk) - kLdA}{A^2}$$

volume $V = AL$, $dV = AdL + LdA$

Dividing equation 2 by equation 1,

$$\frac{dR}{R} = \frac{dL}{L} + \frac{dk}{k} - \frac{dA}{A}$$

3. $$\frac{dR/R}{dL/L} = 1 + \frac{dk/k}{dL/L} - \frac{dA/A}{dL/L}$$

The right-hand side of equation 3 is a function of the nature and the shape of the materials of the strain gauge. Hence, the gauge factor = $\frac{dR/R}{dL/L}$ can be tabulated for given strain gauge material and shape. It is between 2.0 and 3.5 for most materials. Hence, a measurement of dR/R will, when divided by the gauge factor, produce the strain dL/L. Strain gauge meters are calibrated directly in strain when the gauge provided by the manufacturer is used.

Direct measurement of the resistance of the strain gauge does not produce sufficient accuracy for the instrument. Thus, a gauge factor of 2 produces a change in resistance of 2% for each strain of 1%. With a 100-ohm gauge we will be measuring a resistance change of 2 ohms. One configuration for the strain gauge is shown in Figure 3.4.

The Kirchhoff law analysis of the bridge yields the following:

Loop 1: $$V = I_1(R + R)$$

Loop 2: $$V = I_2(R_x + R_s)$$

$$\frac{I_1}{I_2} = \frac{R_x + R_s}{2R}$$

If the rheostat is adjusted so that the meter reads zero:
The potential at loop 1, $E_1 = E_2 =$ the potential at 2

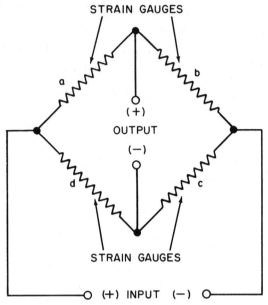

Figure 3.4 Strain gauge circuit. (From B. G. Lipták (ed.) *Instrument Engineers' Handbook* (Vol. I). Philadelphia: Chilton, 1969.)

hence,

$$I_1 R = I_2 R_x$$

and

$$I_1 R = I_2 R_s$$

and by dividing

$$\frac{R}{R} = \frac{R_x}{R_s}$$

The setting of the calibrated rheostat R_x = resistance of gauge R_s. If the calibrated rheostat is a 100-ohm potentiometer, accurate to 0.1%, we could read the 2-ohm resistance of the strain gauge with sufficient accuracy.

TEMPERATURE TRANSDUCERS

The most common temperature transducer is present in every thermostat in every air-conditioned or heater-controlled room or building. It is the bimetallic strip that converts temperature to a displacement. For purposes of continuous monitoring, an electrical signal is desired. Electrical transducers convert temperature to a change in resistance or produce a voltage proportional to the temperature. The former type are resistance thermometers or thermistors, and the latter type is a thermocouple.

RESISTANCE THERMOMETERS

The resistance thermometer operates by converting a change in temperature to a change in electrical resistance. Every material has a temperature coefficient of resistance. The resistance thermometer uses platinum or nickel which has linear reproducible temperature coefficients. Nonmetallic semiconductor-type materials have a negative logarithmic coefficient of resistance. These are called thermistors.

The resistance thermometer using platinum as a sensor defines the International Temperature Scale between −310°F and 1220°F. Platinum is not ordinarily used for industrial or medical applications because of the expense. Nickel wire wound on a mica spool is commonly used. It has a resistance of approximately 100 ohms at 25°C, and a temperature coefficient of 0.0063.

The temperature coefficient of a metal can be expressed by a polynomial:

$$R = R_0(1 + a_1t + a_2t^2 + a_3t^3 + \cdots)$$

where R_0 = resistance in ohms at 0°C
t = temperature in °C

For industrial use the series is truncated after the a_1 term, and the equation becomes

$$R = R_0(1 + at)$$

When the temperature coefficient is given, it is a = 0.0063 that is intended.

THERMISTORS

Since 1835 it has been known that nonmetallic materials have a temperature coefficient. But it was not until 1940 that thermistor materials were subjected to quality control sufficiently rigorous to obtain uniformly reproducible results.

The temperature-resistance characteristic of a thermistor is given by

$$R = R_0 \, e^k$$

where

$$k = b \left(\frac{1}{T} - \frac{1}{T_0} \right)$$

where T is in degrees Kelvin (°K), b = 3400° to 3900°K

As a thermistor is heated, its resistance drops and its current increases. If a thermistor is maintained at constant temperature by a constant source of current, its voltage fluctuates with the amount of heat carried away by the surrounding gas. This principle is used in the thermal conductivity detector used in gas chromatographs. The principle is also used to measure the flow of air in respiration studies.

THERMOCOUPLES

In 1821 Seebeck found that if two different materials formed a junction, a voltage was produced at the junction proportional to its temperature. The voltage formed was very small and could not be utilized until sophisticated secondary devices were developed. The equipment that was developed may be summarized as 1. millivoltmeters, and 2. self-balancing potentiometers.

Recently, with the advent of solid-state circuitry of long-term stability, and the use of the feedback principle to maintain stability of amplifiers, the thermocouples can be connected directly to amplifiers, and reproducible results can be obtained.

The circuit of a thermocouple connected to a millivoltmeter is shown in Figure 3.5. The voltage generated by the thermocouple causes a current to flow through the wire and through the meter coil. The current flow

$$I = V/(R_w + R_m).$$

If R_w and R_m are fixed values, I is proportional to V

$$I = K_R V$$

At the coil, the current produces a magnetic field which causes the meter pointer to rotate in the permanent magnetic field (D'Arsonval movement).

$$F = Bl \ I$$

where Bl = coil constant, and the rotation of the coil is opposed by the torsion of a spring force, so that

$$F = k\theta$$

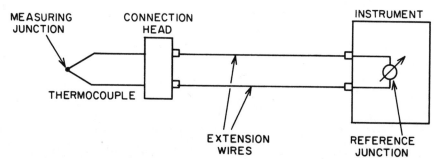

MEASURING JUNCTION   **CONNECTION HEAD**   **INSTRUMENT**

THERMOCOUPLE

EXTENSION WIRES   **REFERENCE JUNCTION**

Figure 3.5 Thermocouple circuit. (From B. G. Lipták (ed.) *Instrument Engineers' Handbook* (Vol. I). Philadelphia: Chilton, 1969.)

where k = spring constant from which

$$\theta = \frac{Bl}{k} I,$$

and the angle is proportional to I which is proportional to V.

OTHER TRANSDUCERS

PRESSURE MEASUREMENTS

The pressure exerted by a fluid is defined in terms of force per unit area, and although it is difficult to compare this quantity with the familiar physiologic blood pressure measurement in millimeters of mercury, let us examine the two types. The force exerted at the bottom of a column of mercury is the weight of that column of mercury. The weight (F) = density × volume and the volume = cross-sectional area × the height. Mathematically,

$$F = dv,$$

and

$$v = hA$$

Therefore,

$$F = dhA$$

or pressure = f/a = dh.

Thus, we refer to a column of mercury 760 mm. high which exerts the same pressure as 1 atmosphere, and 1 atmosphere = 14.7 pounds per square inch pressure.

Mercury has a density of 849 pounds per cubic foot.

$$\frac{760 \text{ mm.}}{25.4 \text{ mm./in.}} = 30 \text{ in. Hg.}$$

$$\frac{849 \text{ lbs./cu. ft.}}{12^3 \text{ cu. in./cu. ft.}} = \frac{849}{1728} \text{ lbs./cu. in.} \times 30 \text{ in.} = 14.7 \text{ lbs./sq. in.}$$

All by way of proving that pressure in mm. Hg really represents a force per unit area.

Pressure measurements are usually obtained from the measurement of the force produced on a standard area. The use of a metal diaphragm provides a reference area to measure the force. The displacement of the diaphragm is the input to an electrical transducer. Thus, pressure is measured by strain gauges and by variable differential transformers.

FLOW MEASUREMENTS

At this point the reader should not be surprised if we could prove that flow measurements can be made with our displacement transducers. In this area, however, physiologic measurements must perforce differ from the process instruments. In measuring flow in a process, the instrument engineer places an orifice in the line and measures the differential pressure drop across the orifice. He thus converts his flow measurement to a pressure measurement, which we have just shown can be measured by a displacement measurement.

Biomedical systems cannot tolerate obstruction. Flow must be measured by a noninvasive method. The biomedical engineer has exercised considerable ingenuity in developing flow measuring devices that do not impede the flow. Two basic principles are used: the magnetic flow meter, and the ultrasonic flow meter.

MAGNETIC FLOW METER

The magnetic flow meter is based on Faraday's law of voltage induction. If a conductor moves perpendicular to a magnetic field, a voltage is induced in a direction mutually perpendicular to the direction of motion of the conductor and the direction of the magnetic field. In Figure 3.6 the conductor is the moving fluid, and the electrodes detect the voltage generated. The magnetic flow meter is used in systems outside the body such as heart-lung machines and artificial kidneys.

ULTRASONIC FLOW METER

The ultrasonic flow meter (Fig. 3.7) requires no invasion of the vessel, but does require invasion of the body so that electrodes can be placed on the surface of the blood vessel. The direct ultrasonic flowmeter utilizes the principle that the vector velocity of the sound in the direction of flow is greater than the vector velocity of the

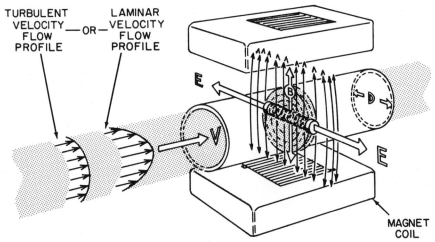

Figure 3.6 Magnetic flow meter. (From B. G. Lipták (ed.) *Instrument Engineers' Handbook* (Vol. I). Philadelphia: Chilton, 1969.)

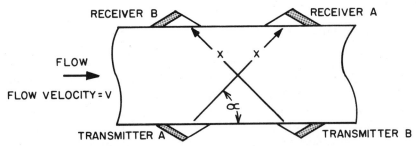

Figure 3.7 Ultrasonic flow meter. (From B. G. Lipták (ed.) *Instrument Engineers' Handbook* (Vol. I). Philadelphia: Chilton, 1969.)

sound perpendicular to the flow by the amount of the flow. Hence, a piezoelectric crystal generates ultrasound of the order of 100 kHz. in frequency. A similar crystal detects the signal a short distance along the blood vessel. Now the procedure is reversed. The downstream crystal is the sender and the upstream crystal the receiver.

$$T_u - T_d = 2dv \frac{\cos \theta}{c^2}$$

where d = distance between crystals
     v = velocity of blood flow
     c = velocity of sound in blood
     T_u = transit time upstream
     T_d = transit time downstream

The Doppler ultrasonic flow meter is based on the principle that ultrasonic vibration radiating from a moving fluid sounds just like audible sound bouncing back from a moving train. The mournful wail that develops when the frequency with which returning sound rises as the train recedes is familiar to a small-town train watcher, and has been introduced to the uninitiated by way of motion pictures and television films. An ultrasonic signal is sent into the blood vessel and detected at its return. The back signal is modulated against the forward signal, and the frequency of modulation is proportional to the rate of blood flow.

RADIATION TRANSDUCERS

Radiation is that form of energy propagated through space in the form of waves. It usually refers to electromagnetic radiation, which may be classified by its frequency as radiofrequency, microwave, infrared, visible, ultraviolet, X-rays, gamma rays, and cosmic rays. The term has been extended to energy emanating from radioactive materials such as alpha, beta, and gamma radiation, although alpha and beta radiation are really particles. Each form of radiation is detected by a unique device peculiar to that frequency. Ultraviolet, visible, and infrared radiation, for example, may be detected by electronic tubes whose cathodes are activated specifically by each type of energy.

Infrared radiation has a heating effect, and its intensity may be detected by a thermopile. Conversely, the temperature of very hot objects may be measured by a radiation pyrometer, which contains a thermopile. The range of radiation pyrometers has been extended downward recently (by cooling the detector) so that they may be applied to skin temperatures. The measurement of the infrared energy emitted by the skin is now used in the detection of breast cancer. The field is called *thermography*.

CHEMICAL TRANSDUCERS

Transducers which respond to the chemical nature of their environment may generally be classified as electromagnetic type or electrochemical type. The electromagnetic type is designed to have a sample flow through a cell interposed between a radiation source and a radiation detector. The chemical in the sample interacts with the specific radiation frequency that characterizes it; if it is detected a signal is generated proportional to the concentration of the material in the sample.

Electrochemical transducers utilize an electrode constructed of material that reacts with the specific ion to be determined, e.g., a silver electrode will react with chloride ion and generate a potential related to the chloride ion concentration. Specific ion electrodes have membranes which permit the diffusion of specific ions only. Inside the electrode membrane is a fluid which allows the ion to activate the proper electrode.

In addition to the two types of transducers just described, there is a great variety of transducers developed for specific applications. The most popular of these is the gas chromatograph, which consists of a small physico-chemical separatory unit (the column) followed by a detector which responds to each component as it emerges from the column. The hot-wire detector is used for the detection of combustible gases. As the gases react on the surface of the detector, they change its temperature, an alteration which changes its resistance which in turn can be detected electrically.

Finally there is a chemical transducer popularly called a "chemist in a box." In this type of unit a complete chemical analysis is automated. A sample is taken, reacted with reagent, separated and passed through a detector, and its composition is recorded or indicated by a digital readout. Automatic blood analyzers are of this nature.

The history and principles of chemical transducers will be discussed in greater detail in Chapters 4 and 5.

DC BRIDGE CIRCUITS

The output of a primary transducer is rarely useful as produced. Some form of secondary transducer is required to prepare the signal for further processing. For example, the strain gauge produces a resistance that varies with the strain. To use this resistance, the gauge must be actuated by an active source of current or voltage to produce a voltage or current drop across the resistance, which in turn can be amplified for use in a terminating display. The thermocouple output has a voltage in the millivolt range. It can be lost if the meter resistance is too high or the leads are too long. A potentiometric bridge provides a varying potential that can be matched against the thermocouple and gives a useful displacement of a pointer or pen as it matches.

We now propose to use circuit analysis theory presented in Chapter 2 to analyze the performance of the bridge networks required to utilize the transducers outlined in this chapter.

Bridge circuits may be classified by the type of electrical parameter they measure (Table 3.1). There are resistance, capacitance, and inductance bridges. There are also bridges to measure voltage and current. There are DC and AC bridges. We shall start with DC bridges to measure resistance and work our way through this three-dimensional maze whose coordinates include types of passive parameters, types of active parameters, and frequency of activation (DC or AC, 1000 Hz., and M-Hz.).

WHEATSTONE BRIDGE

The fundamental bridge circuit for DC resistance is the Wheatstone bridge, shown in Figure 3.8. The excitation of a Wheatstone bridge is by means of a DC voltage. The early Wheatstone bridges were activated by a "Bell battery," now termed an "ignition" battery, which includes doorbells, buzzers, and alarm systems. Most manufacturers call it the "No. 6" and it provides 1½ volts DC.

A Kirchhoff analysis of the bridge shows that with the bridge in balance (current through $G = 0$), a current flows through AX from node 1 and a current flows through BS from node 1. The total current derived from the Kirchhoff current law at node 1 is

$$I = I_{AX} + I_{BS}$$

But since nodes 2 and 3 are at the same potential

1. $\qquad V_{12} = V_{13} \qquad I_{AX}A = I_{BS}B$

2. $\qquad V_{24} = V_{34} \qquad I_{AX}X = I_{BS}S$

TABLE 3.1 PRIMARY TRANSDUCERS AND THEIR BRIDGES

Primary Transducer	Bridge
Displacement Transducers	
linear resistance	resistance bridge
differential transformer	reluctance bridge
variable-inductance	inductance bridge
capacitive transducer	capacitance bridge
piezoelectric transducer	charge amplifier
flapper-nozzle transducer	pressure transmitter
Force Transducers	
spring balance	linear resistance
elastic transducers	see displacement
strain gauge	strain gauge bridge
Temperature Transducers	
bimetallic strip	relay
resistance thermometer	resistance bridge
thermistor	special amplifier
thermocouples	potentiometric bridge millivolt meter
Pressure Transducers	
strain gauge	strain gauge bridge
elastic transducers	see displacement
Flow Measurements	
magnetic flow meter	voltage amplifier
ultrasonic flow meter	special amplifier detector
Radiation Transducers	
thermal radiation	thermopile
radiofrequency radiation	tuned circuit
microwave radiation	klystron tube
infrared radiation	bolometer
visible radiation	photocell
ultraviolet radiation	ultraviolet phototube
X-radiation	Geiger-Müller tube
	photographic plate
gamma rays	gamma ray spectrometer
cosmic rays	ionization chamber
alpha radiation	proportional counter
beta radiation	scintillation counter
	proportional counter
ionization chamber	proportional counter
Geiger-Müller tube scintillation	amplifier-counter-scaler register
Chemical Transducers	
electromagnetic type	
electrochemical type	VTVM amplifiers (pH meters)
gas chromatograph	peak picker-recorder
"chemist in a box"	electromotive or electrochemical type output
combustible gas	hot-wire bridge (filament)

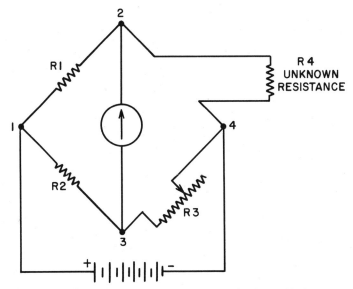

Figure 3.8 Wheatstone bridge. (From B. G. Lipták (ed.) *Instrument Engineers' Handbook* (Vol. II). Philadelphia: Chilton, 1970.)

dividing 2 by 1

$$\frac{X}{A} = \frac{S}{B}$$

or

3. $$X = \frac{SA}{B}$$

If X is the resistance of a strain gauge, its value can be determined from the known values of A, B, and S in equation 3. The configuration shown in Figure 3.8 will be valid for one value of X only. To extend the range of the bridge we have two alternatives: 1) adjust S to balance the bridge, or 2) calibrate the deflection of the meter for changes in values of X. The first choice is called the Null method and the second the Deflection method.

Null Method—Slidewire Bridges

In the slidewire bridge (Fig. 3.9), resistors A and B are replaced with a continuous wire of uniform cross-sectional area. Since

$$R = kL/A$$

and since k and A are constant, the resistance (R) is proportional to the length. In practice, the slidewire is a wound coil with a sliding contact to increase its resistivity per unit length, made of manganin to reduce the effect of temperature.

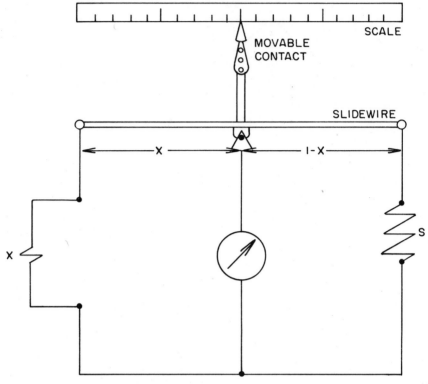

Figure 3.9 Adjustable Wheatstone bridge.

At balance

$$\frac{X}{S} = \frac{x}{1-x} \quad \text{or} \quad X = \frac{Sx}{1-x}$$

S = adjustable slider which is moved to obtain the value of resistance $x/(1-x)$ at the adjustable ratio arm, adjustable to $(x|1-x) = 0.1, 1.0, 10.0$, etc.

The procedure just described can be carried out automatically by the device shown in Figure 3.10.

Deflection Bridge

For the measurement of rapidly changing signals the bridge balancing method would miss the dynamics of the signal. To observe the actual progress of the signal, the unbalanced bridge method is used. The bridge is balanced at the operating point as already outlined. With the dynamic signal coming in, however, the bridge is not re-balanced to match the signal, and the galvanometer is allowed to indicate the change in signal.

Computation of the current flowing through the meter can be per-

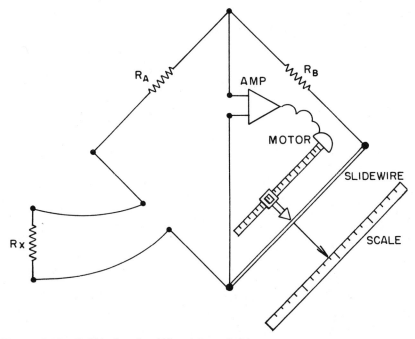

Figure 3.10 Self-balancing Wheatstone bridge.

formed by use of Thevenin's theorem. A portion of a network can be replaced by an equivalent voltage source and an equivalent series resistance (Fig. 3.11). The network is opened at two terminals, and the equivalent voltage source is equal to the voltage that can be measured at those terminals with no other outside connections. The

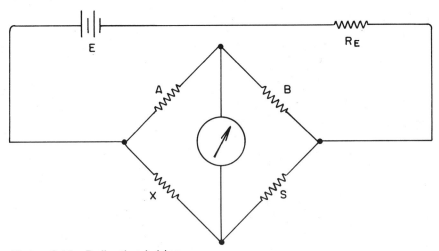

Figure 3.11 Deflection bridge.

series resistance is similarly the resistance between those two terminals with all internal voltages inactive.

The Thevenin voltage would be

$$E_m = \frac{E(AS - BX)}{R_E(A + B + X + S) + (A + B)(X + S)}$$

To calculate the Thevenin resistance assume

$$E = 0$$

$$R_{th} = \frac{AB}{A + B} + \frac{XS}{X + S}$$

The current through the meter, when connected, can be calculated by Ohm's law, written on the total resistance $R_{th} + R_m$ and the total voltage E_m.

$$i_m = \frac{E_m}{R_{th} + R_m}$$

POTENTIOMETRIC BRIDGES

The term *potentiometer* in this connection means to "meter potential." If a potential source is connected to a uniform resistance wire, as in Figure 3.12, the location of any point on the slidewire will represent a potential point above ground. If E_B is the voltage of the battery, when $x = 1.0$ (full scale), we should tap off E_B volts; when $x = 0$, we should tap off zero volts; and when $x = 0.5$, we should tap off $0.5E_B$ volts. For the voltmeter to read correctly, its internal resistance must be 100 or 1000× the resistance of the slidewire.

$$R_m = 1000 \ R_s$$

If we were going to compare an unknown potential with the known

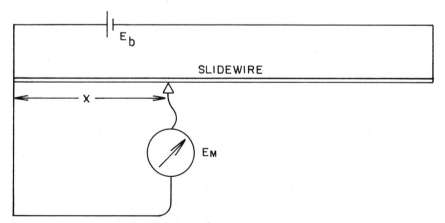

Figure 3.12 Potentiometric bridge.

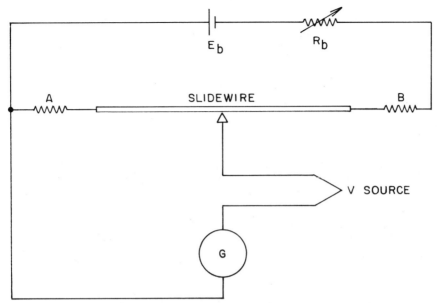

Figure 3.13   Variable zero-variable range bridge.

potential across the slidewire we would first calibrate the slidewire. A known electromotive force (e.m.f.) (standard cell) will be connected at the sample point, and the battery current adjusted by R_b until the null meter reads zero. If the unknown e.m.f. is now connected and the slider moved until the null indicator reads zero, the calibrated slidewire will provide a reading of the e.m.f. of the unknown potential.

In a practical potentiometer it becomes necessary to be able to adjust the zero and the range of the slidewire. For example, suppose one wanted to indicate 50°F to 150°F with an iron-constantin thermocouple. With a reference junction at 32°F the thermocouple will generate 0.50 mv. at the lower limit and 3.41 mv. at the upper limit. Hence, we would like a potentiometer bridge with a zero at 0.50 mv. and a range of $3.41 - 0.50 = 2.91$ mv. To do so the configuration in Figure 3.13 is used.

Analysis of the circuit in Figure 3.13 yields the following information:

The potential drop across A is $e_0 = iA$

The potential drop across the slidewire $e_r = iS$

Hence,

$$e_0/e_r = A/S$$

and the size of the resistor A is

$$A = (e_0/e_r)S$$

The potential drop across the resistor B

$$E - (e_0 + e_r) = iB$$

shows that the size of the resistor B must be

$$B = \frac{E}{e_r} S - \left(\frac{e_0}{e_r} + 1\right) S$$

Resistor A adjusts the zero point and resistor B adjusts the range of the bridge.

AC BRIDGE CIRCUITS

To measure capacitance and inductance, AC bridge circuits are required. These bridges can also be used in resistance measurements, and they are used when DC would polarize the measuring device (as in electrochemical cells, or if thermal electromotive forces were present).

If to each resistor in a Wheatstone bridge are added a capacitance and an inductance, the impedance of each arm replaces the resistance in the bridge balance equation:

1.
$$\frac{Z_1}{Z_2} = \frac{Z_3}{Z_4}$$

The complex impedance is expressed as

$$Z = R + jwL \text{ for inductance}$$

and

$$Z = R + 1/jwC \text{ for capacitance.}$$

The impedance is a vector with magnitude and direction (Fig. 3.14). The magnitude

$$|Z| = \sqrt{R^2 + w^2L^2}$$

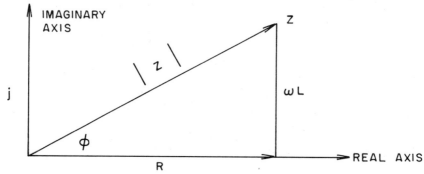

Figure 3.14 Relationship between impedance and resistance.

and the angle

$$\phi = \tan^{-1} (wL/R)$$

Impedance can also be expressed as

$$Z = |Z| (\cos \phi + j \sin \phi)$$

or if we note that

$$e^{j\phi} = \cos \phi + j \sin \phi,$$

then

$$Z = |Z| e^{j\phi}$$

Thus when two impedances are multiplied

$$Z = Z_1 Z_2 = |Z_1| \cdot |Z_2| \ e^{j\phi_1} \cdot e^{j\phi_2} = |Z| \ e^{j(\phi_1 + \phi_2)}) = |Z| \ e^{j\phi},$$

the magnitudes are multiplied

$$|Z| = |Z_1| \cdot |Z_2|$$

and the phase angles are added

$$\phi = \phi_1 + \phi_2$$

In the case of the Wheatstone bridge, when it is at balance

$$\frac{Z_1}{Z_2} = \frac{Z_3}{Z_4}$$

$$\frac{|Z_1|}{|Z_2|} = \frac{|Z_3|}{|Z_4|}$$

and

$$\phi_1 - \phi_2 = \phi_3 - \phi_4$$

Physically, this means that to balance the bridge two adjustments are required, one for the magnitude and one for the phase. Since the factors are interrelated, the adjustment must be by trial-and-error until balance is achieved.

Figure 3.15 shows A) a simple Wheatstone bridge with resistors only but AC actuated, B) a Wheatstone bridge measuring the impedance of an unknown by a series-capacitance comparison, C) a Wheatstone bridge measuring an unknown impedance by a parallel-capacitance comparison, and D) a configuration known as a Maxwell bridge. In the simple AC Wheatstone bridge the only difference from the DC bridge is the detector. Note that a pair of earphones is shown as the detector. If we use 1000 Hz. as the actuating signal, we can hear this tone on the earphones. When the bridge is balanced the tone is at minimum intensity. An oscilloscope can be used to display the

AC signal. R_3 is adjusted until the tone or signal is at minimum intensity. Then $R_x = R_3R_2/R_1$. With R_2/R_1 known and R_3 readable from its scale, R_x can be determined.

If the unknown impedance is capacitive, circuit B of Figure 3.15 may be used. The solution of this circuit by our circuit rules is

1.
$$\frac{Z_1}{Z_3} = \frac{Z_2}{Z_4}$$

$$\frac{R_1}{R_3 - jX_{c_3}} = \frac{R_2}{R_x - jX_{c_x}}$$

Invert to bring imaginaries into numerator and divide

$$\frac{R_3}{R_1} - \frac{jX_{c_3}}{R_1} = \frac{R_x}{R_2} - \frac{jX_{c_x}}{R_2}$$

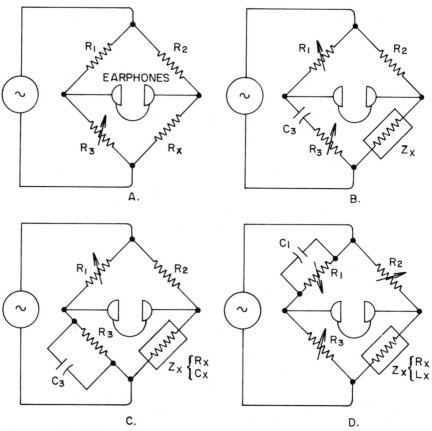

Figure 3.15 AC Wheatstone bridges. *A*, Simple bridge for measurement; *B*, Bridge for measuring series resistance-capacitance; *C*, Bridge for measuring parallel resistance-capacitance; *D*, A Maxwell bridge for inductance.

separating the real parts from the imaginary parts

$$\frac{R_3}{R_1} = \frac{R_x}{R_2} \quad \text{and} \quad \frac{X_{c_3}}{R_1} = \frac{X_{c_x}}{R_2}$$

from which

$$Rx = \frac{R_3 R_2}{R_1} \quad \text{and} \quad \frac{X_{c_x}}{X_{c_3}} = \frac{R_2}{R_1} = \frac{wC_x}{wC_3} = \frac{C_x}{C_3}$$

and we can solve for $C_x = \dfrac{C_3 R_2}{R_1}$.

   Similarly the following results will be obtained from the other bridges:

For the Parallel Capacitance bridge,

$$R_x = R_3 R_2/R_1$$

$$C_x = C_3 R_2/R_1$$

For the Maxwell bridge (used when Z is an inductance)

$$R_x = R_2 R_3/R_1$$

$$L_x = R_2 R_3 C_1$$

Balance is achieved by alternate adjustments of R_1 and R_2. Other configurations of capacitance and Inductance bridge are shown in Fig. 3.16. The Hays bridge (Resistor R_1 is in series with C_1) is a series-capacitance version of the Maxwell bridge.

$$L_x = R_2 R_3 C_1/(1 + w^2 C_1^2 R_1^2)$$

$$R_x = w^2 C_1^2 R_1 R_2 R_3/(1 + w^2 C_1^2 R_1^2)$$

The Owen bridge can be used for measuring inductance of a coil under DC excitation.

$$L_x = C_1 R_2 R_3$$

$$R_x = C_1 R_2 (1/C_3)$$

The Heaviside mutual inductance bridge can be used to measure the mutual inductance between two windings if the self-inductance of one winding is known.

$$R_2 R_3 = R_1 R_4$$

$$M = R_2 L_3 - R_1 L_4/(R_1 + R_2)$$

The Wein bridge is used to measure frequency

$$w^2 = 1/R_3 R_4 C_3 C_4$$

or, since $f = w/2\pi$

$$f = \frac{1}{2\pi} \sqrt{R_3 R_4 C_3 C_4}$$

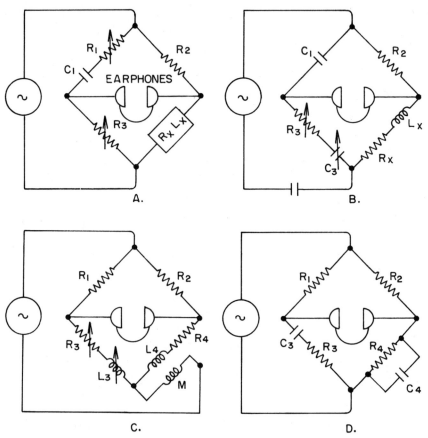

Figure 3.16 Capacitance and inductance bridges. *A,* Hays capacitance bridge; *B,* Owens inductance bridge; *C,* Heaviside mutual inductance bridge; *D,* Wein frequency bridge.

SUMMARY

Electrical transducers convert a primary measurement to an electrical signal. Displacement transducers produce changes in resistance, capacitance, or inductance in electrical circuits. Force transducers move elastic elements to produce a displacement which is then converted to electrical signals. The strain gauge is connected to an elastic element to provide a change in resistance of the wire with strain. Temperature transducers produce a change in resistance with temperature, or thermocouples produce a voltage based on the temperature. Pressure measurements produce a force which is transduced into an electrical signal.

Flow measurements in industrial processes are made to produce pressure drops by placing obstructions in the line. This cannot be done in biomedical systems, hence special methods have been developed like magnetic flow meters and Doppler ultrasonic meters.

Radiation transducers are available for every electromagnetic frequency range. Chemical transducers produce change in radiation absorption, or use electrochemical electrodes, a gas chromatograph, or an automated chemical reaction.

EXERCISES

1. Given the following thermoelectric potentials, what would be the potential of each of the following thermocouples with a reference junction at 32°F. (0°C.): a. iron-constantin at 100°F.; b. copper-constantin at 50°F.; c. chromel-alumel at 100°C.; d. platinum-rhodium at 50°C.; e. antimony-constantin at −100°C.

Thermoelectric Potentials (microvolts per °C.)
referred to platinum at 0°C.

iron	18.5
constantin	−35.0
copper	6.5
chromel	25.0
antimony	47.0
rhodium	6.0
alumel	−15.0

2. A simple Wheatstone bridge has arms with the following values: R_1 = 100 ohms, R_2 = 50 ohms, R_3 = 101 ohms. Calculate the value of R_4 to obtain balance.

3. What would be the error of the reading of the potentiometer in Figure 3.12 if the slidewire has a resistance of 100 ohms and the meter has a resistance of 1000 ohms? Calculate the error at low potential, midscale, and high potential if E_b is a 1.0 volt battery.

4. What would be the error of the bridge in Figure 3.15 if it were energized by 60-cycle 100-volt current, and the resistance measured (100 ohms) had a capacitance of 1 farad associated with its windings? Assume $R_1 = R_2 = 100$ ohms.

5. What would be the settings of R_3 and C_3 if the coil described in problem 3 were measured by the bridge in Figure 3.15B, modified so that the capacitor C_3 is variable and the resistor $R_1 = R_2 = 100$ ohms?

6. What would be the settings of R_3 and C_3 of the Owens bridge in Figure 3.16B if the unknown transformer winding had a resistance of 1.0 ohm and an inductance of 100 millihenries. Assume R_2 and C_1 values to give midscale readings.

General Literature Cited and References

Alt, F. Advances in Bioengineering and Medicine. New York: Plenum, 1966.

Beckwith, T. G., and Buck, N. L. Mechanical Measurements. Reading, Mass.: Addison-Wesley, 1969.

Considine, D. M. Process Instruments and Controls Handbook. New York: McGraw-Hill, 1957.

Lipták, B. G. (editor) Instrument Engineers' Handbook (Vol. 1). Philadelphia: Chilton, 1969.

Minnar, E. J. (editor) ISA Transducer Compendium. New York: Plenum, 1963.

Norton, H. N. Handbook of Transducers for Electronic Measuring Systems. Englewood Cliffs: Prentice-Hall, 1969.

Chapter 4

Physiologic Measurements

PHYSIOLOGY is the systematic study of the functioning of living systems. Cybernetics, the study of communication and control in both living and man-made systems, has made every physiologist a systems analyst. The human system, says the systems analyst, is a structure of subsystems, each of which can be broken down into simpler component systems, until we arrive at the most elemental system, the cell. We shall see that even the cell can be broken down into its constituents, the organelles (the organs in the cell). Among these are the nucleus, which contains the genes (DNA), the organizing molecule of the cell; the cytoplasm, the plasma inside the cell, which itself contains the endoplasmic reticulum (the chemical factory of the cell); and the mitochondria, the energy source of the cell.

THE CELL

The cell is observed by the classic instrument of biological observation, the light microscope. With it we can observe the structures of the cell, but not their function. The electron microscope extended our vision to the microelements or ultrastructures of the cell—the organelles and inclusions. The electrical and chemical signals inside the cell only became observable, however, when the microelectrode was developed, and radioactive tracers became available to study chemical compositional changes.

The microelectrode is a glass tube drawn to a point less than 1 micron (1×10^{-6} meters) in diameter, and hollow at the tip. By a phenomenal technique the tube is filled with a solution of potassium chloride, which conducts the potential from the cell to an internal silver or platinum wire. In addition to the measuring electrode inside the cell, a second reference electrode is located outside the cell, at a neutral position. When properly performed, the technique measures a potential of −90 mv. immediately after the cell wall is penetrated.*

The Nernst equation is used by physical chemists to calculate the potential generated by a concentration gradient between solutions:

$$E = \frac{RT}{nF} \ln \frac{[C_a]_1}{[C_a]_2}$$

where E = potential in millivolts

R = gas constant (which converts temperature to energy units)

F = Faraday constant (96,500 coulombs per chemical equivalent)

n = number of chemical equivalents per atom

$[C_a]_1, [C_a]_2$ = symbols for concentration of atom a in solutions 1 and 2

T = temperature in °K

At the body temperature of 37°C, the factor $RT/F = 61$ mv. (including the factor 2.303 needed to convert the natural log ln to $\log_{10}$). At the concentrations given in Table 1.1 the potential E is essentially equal to the −90 mv. observed by the microelectrode.

If we look at the concentrations in Table 1.1, we see a phenomenon that cannot be explained by physical chemistry. The potassium concentration is higher inside the cell and lower outside the cell. Hence, potassium normally tends to diffuse out, whereas sodium which has a higher concentration outside the cell and a lower concentration inside the cell tends to diffuse in.

The physiologist explains this anomaly by postulating the presence of a *sodium pump*. An active mechanism exists in the membrane of the cell which pumps sodium ions out, thus leaving a shortage of positive charges inside the cell which helps to keep the potassium ions in.

The nonequilibrium condition is maintained by the pump, and the ionic imbalance can be measured in terms of the resting potential of the cell. Hence, just to maintain itself at rest, the cell is working.

NERVE CELLS AND SIGNAL TRANSMISSION

The fundamental element of the nervous system is the neuron, or nerve cell (Fig. 4.1). In order to perform its function (the transmission of signals), the nerve cell has many short (input) arms called dendrites

---

* At this point we do not mention the difficult instrumentation problems involved in measuring this biolectric potential, some of which will be discussed later.

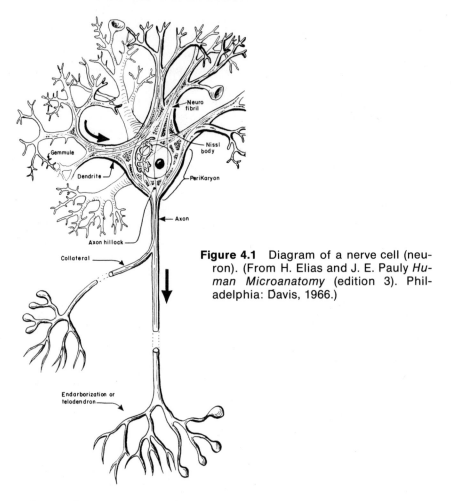

Figure 4.1 Diagram of a nerve cell (neuron). (From H. Elias and J. E. Pauly *Human Microanatomy* (edition 3). Philadelphia: Davis, 1966.)

and a single output arm called the axon. Some axons are insulated by fatty tissue called myelin. At the end of the axon the nerve divides into many parts, each one of which may contain an end plate which can transmit the nervous signal to a muscle. Signals are transmitted from neuron to neuron, or from neuron to muscle at the synapse (synaptic junction). At the discontinuity, a transmitter substance is generated by the nerve cell which chemically activates the input to the next cell.

How does the nervous signal move along the neuron? If a micro-electrode is placed inside the neuron, a signal is obtained. This signal can be shown to be the result of interference with the normal sodium pump. If the pump stops, sodium will diffuse into the nerve cell, increasing the potential from −70 mv.* to more than 20 mv. If the normal

---

* The resting potential of nerve tissue is −70 mv.; that of muscle cells (which was used in the preceding example) is −90 mv.

sodium concentration gradient prevailed, a potential of 60 mv. would be obtained. But before that level is reached, the sodium influx stops. Also, during this period of normal diffusion, some of the potassium from inside the cell diffuses out, decreasing the internal positive potential. The action potential signal then reverses itself as the sodium is pumped out and overshoots in the negative direction to -75 mv., after which it slowly returns to its resting potential of -70 mv. The depletion of potassium from inside the cell is the reason for this latter overshoot. As the potassium diffuses slowly back into the cell, the internal potential returns to its reference value.

MUSCLE CELLS AND POWER PRODUCTION

Muscle tissue consists of individual fiber-like cells held together by connective tissue. Each individual fiber has the ability to contract when stimulated from its resting potential of -90 mv.

No scale is shown for the tension developed in the muscle, for this will depend, among other factors, on the initial length of the muscle fiber. If a second action potential is produced before the muscle has relaxed, the second contraction wave is superimposed on the first. If the stimulus is repeated rapidly enough, a smooth continued response is obtained which is called *tetanus*.

The measurement of action potentials of individual muscles is useful in the study of normal and pathologic muscle conditions. The record of the action potential of a muscle is called an electromyogram (EMG).

The action potential of *cardiac muscle* has a long refractory period. This difference in response from that of skeletal muscle means that repeated stimuli received while the muscle is contracting will not affect the muscle. The muscle will proceed through its entire contraction — relaxation cycle before it will contract again. Tetanus is therefore not possible for cardiac muscle, which is fortunate, since cardiac muscle would not pump while subjected to tetanus.

The response of *smooth muscle* to enervation may vary from a response similar to that of skeletal muscle to one similar to cardiac muscle. Depolarization is slow and produces a prepotential stage prior to the action potential stage.

ENERGY IN THE CELL

The principal power plant of the cell consists of the mitochondria. Within these organelles adenosine triphosphate (ATP) is manufactured from adenosine diphosphate (ADP) by the reaction of oxygen with nutrients prepared by the cellular cytoplasm. The reaction product, carbon dioxide, diffuses out of the cell into the blood vessels to be eliminated by the lungs. The detailed chemistry of the Krebs cycle which takes place in the mitochondria can be studied in any biochemical or medical physiology text. The ATP is used in the cell for 1) generation of the action potential, when required (here the connection is indirect, too; the ATP is used to operate the sodium pump.); 2) production of contraction in muscle tissue, when required; and 3) synthesis of chemical compounds in the cell, e.g., the manufacture of DNA in the ribosomes. When so used, the ATP is converted to ADP, which returns to the mitochondria for reactivation to ATP by the use of more oxygen and nutrients and the production of more carbon dioxide.

MEMORY IN THE CELL—DNA

The same genes that control heredity also control the continuous functioning of each cell. The genes constitute the memory of the cell. As a result of the application of the electron microscope, X-ray diffraction studies, and biochemical analysis and synthesis, it is known that the genes are composed of DNA, deoxyribonucleic acid. These genes contain amino acids arranged in a definite configuration which may be likened to code words. In order to multiply, the DNA molecule uses ribonucleic acid (RNA). It forms various types of RNA, e.g., messenger RNA, soluble RNA, and others. Upon formation, messenger RNA carries the genetic code to the endoplasmic reticulum for formation of other proteins. Soluble RNA, on the other hand, finds the proper amino acids and brings them to this site. As each type of amino acid is delivered, the messenger matrix forms them into the protein molecule.

THE NERVOUS SYSTEM

Cyberneticists in their study of communication and control in the human system have learned techniques which they have applied directly to the design of synthetic systems, e.g., the digital computer. The language of the systems engineer is now patterned after the language of the neurophysiologist. The systems engineer studies topics like reflexive control, adaptive control, optimizing control, learning systems, and pattern recognition, all of which are functions of the nervous system as well as of a properly designed control system.

It will be useful at this point to review the principle of feedback control and the terminology of the control engineer, especially to see how these factors parallel the structure and functioning of the human nervous system.

FEEDBACK CONTROL AND REFLEXIVE ACTION

The feedback control loop can be described by a block diagram as a technique for controlling a process (Fig. 4.2). One of the variables of

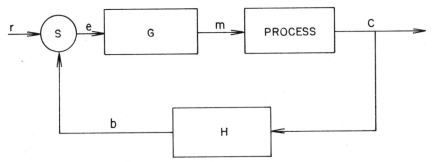

Figure 4.2 Canonical form of feedback control.

the process is selected for measurement (c) and one is selected for manipulation (m). A transducer (H) converts the measured variable to a useful signal (b). The comparator (S) compares the measured signal with the desired signal (r) to produce an error signal (e). The error signal now becomes the actuating signal for the controller (G) which modifies the manipulated signal (m) in a manner to place the process under control.

We can see how the same principle is used to control the action of picking up a pencil. When you move your hand to pick up a pencil, you don't *know* what you are doing. You have learned a response stored in the nerve connections of your spinal cord, which sends signals to the proper muscles when your brain tells this center that your hand must move. This procedure is known by the control engineer as a "servomechanism," a control system designed to meet a moving target. Your eye is the transducer that senses the position of the pencil (target). This sensed position is the reference for the control action to be taken. The actual position of your hand is sensed by kinesthetic receptors in the muscles of your hand (which makes it possible for you to close your eyes and touch the spot which is the target). Your eyes are also sending signals about your hand's position, which you may or may not use as a correction signal to the kinesthetic signal.

Synapses in the spinal cord respond to the signal e to produce pulses of action potential to the required muscles, which contract on command to move the hand. The biological sensors in the muscle spindles send fresh signals, and the tour around the loop is repeated, until, when e becomes zero, no actuating signal appears at the nerve center, and no additional muscle motion is demanded.

Figure 4.3 shows what control engineers call *on-off control*. A bolus of food is moving along the small intestine. A stretch receptor in the small intestine senses the bolus and "turns on the switch," which activates the smooth muscle to contract, pushing the food along its way by peristaltic action to digestion and excretion.

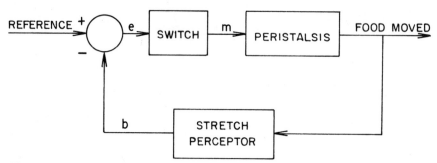

Figure 4.3 Reflexive control of visceral muscles.

THE AUTONOMIC NERVOUS SYSTEM

A third term used by control engineers to define a control action is regulation. A *regulator* is a feedback control system that maintains a fixed level of some variable within the system. In the internal environment of the body many such regulators exist, maintaining the temperature of the body, the composition of the blood, and the pressure of the blood. All of these regulators form part of the autonomic nervous system (ANS), which controls the involuntary functions of the body.

As for most of the important functions of the body, the ANS consists of two partially antagonistic divisions, the sympathetic nervous system and the parasympathetic nervous system. Table 4.1 outlines the antagonistic action of the ANS.

Sympathetic action increases the heart rate, produces sweat, releases glucose required for quick energy, dilates the pupils, and prepares the body for danger. Parasympathetic action stimulates the internal glands for digesting food, decreases the heart rate, relaxes blood vessels, and prepares the body for rest and relaxation.

The autonomic reflexes are the regulatory functions of the ANS.— they maintain homeostasis. One of its regulatory functions is the

TABLE 4.1 ANTAGONISTIC ACTION OF THE AUTONOMIC NERVOUS SYSTEM

Organ	Sympathetic Action	Parasympathetic Action
Heart	Increase in rate and force	Decrease in rate and force
Blood vessels	Constriction	Dilation
Clot rate	Increase	No effect
Glucose	Increase	No effect
Pupil of eye	Dilation	Contraction
Glands:		
Tears, gastric, pancreatic	Constriction	Stimulation
Sweat	Stimulation	No effect

maintenance of blood pressure. When pressure receptors located in the carotid body and aorta become overstretched by increased pressure, a signal sent to the brainstem inhibits sympathetic activity, which reduces heart force and rate and decreases blood pressure. Another control involves digestion. The odor and sight of food stimulates a section of the brain to send parasympathetic signals to the salivary glands and to the digestive glands of the stomach.

The hypothalamus is the control center in the brainstem for the integration of sympathetic and parasympathetic activities, and for the control of the involuntary functions of the body. Centers in the hypothalamus have been identified for the regulation of heart pressure and rate, body temperature, body water control, gastrointestinal control, endocrine functions, and control of excitement and rage. The hypothalamus also generates signals such as thirst and hunger.

THE BRAIN AND COGITATIVE ACTION

Enough is known about certain portions of the brain to be able to understand their functions with respect to the cogitative activities of the human organism. Such activities include the state of being awake, the technique of directing attention to specific areas in our conscious minds, and the processes of thinking, remembering, and learning. A bit of anatomy of the brain will be useful here.

The *cerebral cortex* is the surface area of the brain. It has been mapped by means of electrodes during neurological surgery, and by observing large numbers of patients with destroyed cortical regions. It is the motor control and primary sensory region of the brain.

The *reticular activating system* is located at the base of the brain. Signals from the body pass through the spinal cord and this area to enter the brain. This system is believed to control the degree of central nervous system activity and the state of wakefulness and attention. When an animal is asleep, the reticular activating system is dormant. But almost any sensory signal can activate the system. Pain, signals from the muscles, and visual or auditory signals can activate the system.

Brain wave activity from the surface of the brain seems to be related to mental activity. Cerebration tends to produce asynchronous pulses in the neurons of the brain, but brain waves must originate from simultaneous firing of many neurons in the brain, and therefore must be associated with a low level of cerebration.

The electroencephalograph (EEG) records four types of brain waves characterized by different frequencies and amplitudes. The *alpha* waves occur at a frequency of 8 to 13 cycles per second with an amplitude of 50 microvolts. They appear in the normal subject while he is awake, quiet, and resting. They disappear in sleep, or when the awake subject directs his thoughts to a specific matter.

Beta waves occur at frequencies between 14 and 50 cycles per second. They occur during tension or intense activation of the central nervous system.

Delta waves have frequencies from 3.5 cycles per second to 1 cycle every 3 seconds. They can occur in the cortex independent of activities in the other parts of the brain. They are found in states of deep sleep, infancy, and serious brain disease.

Theta waves with frequencies between 4 and 7 cycles per second occur in adults under emotional stress or frustration.

The basic rhythm of the EEG seems to increase with the degree of cerebral activity. Delta waves occur in sleep, stupor, and surgical procedures; theta waves are found in infants; alpha waves occur during relaxation; and beta waves occur during periods of intense activity. During epilepsy of the grand mal type, intense cerebral activity takes place, and the EEG is even more rapid.

The EEG is used to diagnose epilepsy, brain lesions, and subdural hematomas (blood clots below the outermost membrane of brain and spinal cord).

The theory of memory is in a state of transition. The synapse theory held that synapses were locked into configurations that produced memory responses like the binary condition of core spaces in a digital computer. But with the discovery of short-term and long-term memory it is now believed that the synapse condition may be responsible for short-term memory, but that long-term memory is associated with modification of the DNA code in particular neurons.

BIOLOGICAL TRANSDUCERS

Since the sensory nerve endings detect a sensory stimulus and convert it to a standard internal signal, they can be properly called biological transducers. The standard signal is the action potential firing of an adjacent neuron. Neurons will either fire an action potential or remain inert. The details of the action potential have already been outlined. It has an initial (refractory) period during which it will not fire despite being restimulated, after which it will refire if stimulated.

The sensory receptor continues to emit a stimulating potential to the adjacent neuron, as long as the receptor itself is stimulated. This continued signal produces a signal of pulses along the nerve trunk, whose number is a function of the intensity of the stimulus. That this function is approximately logarithmic has caused the transducer engineer to use logarithmic units (decibels) to describe signals (like sound) detectable by human beings.

The perception of a sensory signal takes place in the brain. All signals along the nerve trunks are alike, pulses of action potential. Each type of biological signal is transmitted to a specific area in the brain,

TABLE 4.2 SENSORY NERVE ENDINGS

Stimulus	Receptor
Mechanical	
touch	Meissner's corpuscle
pain	free nerve endings
pressure	Pacinian corpuscle
kinesthetic	muscle spindles
sound vibrations	cochlea
acceleration and balance	semicircular canals
stretch of lungs and heart	pressure receptors
Thermal	
cold	Krause's end bulb
warmth	corpuscle of Ruffini
Chemical	
taste	taste buds
smell	olfactory cells
oxygen levels in blood	carotid body, aortic body
Electromagnetic	
light	rods and cones in retina

and is recognized by the brain by the location of its terminus. Thus, touch receptors in the skin terminate in touch perception areas of the brain, and taste receptors in the mouth terminate in taste perception areas in the brain. A tabulation of receptors is given in Table 4.2.

THE CIRCULATORY SYSTEM

Fluid flow through living tissue follows the same laws as fluid flow through a rigid pipe, but the elasticity of the living tissue produces much different results. For example, when the veins receive increased blood flow, they relax and absorb the volume, increasing the blood pressure very slightly. When a blood vessel is severed, the veins can contract to maintain normal blood circulation even though 25% of the blood is lost; the blood vessel can contract and expand. The capillary is a leaky pipe, allowing nutrients to flow into the tissues and feed the cells. The heart is quite different from an ordinary pump. It runs on its own fluid, the coronary blood circulation which provides the nutrients required to operate the heart muscle.

Hemodynamics is the study of the particular kind of fluid dynamics that applies to the blood. Electrocardiography is the study of the electrical signals associated with running the pump. A study of the blood vessels and the heart is necessary for the understanding of the measurements and control processes involved in blood pressure and blood chemistry, and the signals used for intensive care and coronary care units. In fact, electrical signals from the heart form the major inputs to the electronic monitoring system used in most hospitals.

FLUID FLOW THROUGH LIVING TISSUES

The variables for fluid flow through living tissue are analogous to the variables described in Chapter 2 concerning current flow through electrical circuits. From Table 4.3 the complete story of hemodynamics can be outlined.

The equation of continuity states that the quantity of blood pumped by the heart is equal to the quantity that passes through the systemic circulation, and is equal to the quantity that flows through the pulmonary circulation. (We are omitting consideration of the small volume of coronary flow at this time.) For solid pipes, the equation of continuity states that

$$\text{Flow} = \text{velocity} \times \text{cross-sectional area}$$

The equation of flow states that the flow through any container is equal to the driving force divided by the resistance. The driving force for flow is pressure differential, hence the equation for flow is

1.
$$F = \frac{P_1 - P_2}{R}, \text{ or}$$

$$\text{Flow} = \frac{\text{driving force}}{\text{resistance}} = \frac{\text{difference in pressure}}{\text{flow resistance}}$$

The *resistance* for a flow system is defined by Poiseuille's law for a viscous fluid:

2.
$$v = \frac{(P_1 - P_2)r^2}{8\mu L}$$

where v = velocity of flow in cm./per sec.
$P_1 - P_2$ = the pressure gradient in cm. of the fluid flowing
r = radius of vessel in cm.
μ = viscosity in poises
L = length of vessel in cm.

TABLE 4.3 CURRENT VOLTAGE ANALOGY OF FLUID FLOW

Electrical variable	quantity (coulombs)	current (amperes)	potential (volts)	resistance (ohms, volts/amp)	capacitance (farads, coul./volt)
Hemodynamic variable	volume (ml.)	flow (ml./min.)	pressure (mm. Hg)	peripheral resistance units (press./ flow)	compliance (vol./press)

TABLE 4.4 TYPICAL PERIPHERAL RESISTANCE UNITS

Circulation	PRU
Systemic	
strongly constricted	4.0
normal	1.0
greatly dilated	0.25
Pulmonary	
strongly constricted (diseased)	1.0
normal	0.09
during extreme exercise	0.02

By the equation of continuity

3.
$$F = v\pi r^2 = \frac{(P_1 - P_2)\pi r^4}{8\mu L}$$

comparing with equation 1.

4.
$$R = \frac{8\mu L}{\pi r^4}$$

Therefore, the resistance to flow is directly proportional to the viscosity and length and inversely proportional to the radius of the vessel to the fourth power. Blood is different from water due to the presence of blood solids and cells. The major effect on the viscosity is the hematocrit,* or red cell content of the blood. Water has a viscosity of 1.002 centipoises at reference temperature. Compared with this, plasma has a viscosity of 1.5 centipoises, and normal blood, 3.5 centipoises at hematocrit of 40. At hematocrit of 70, the viscosity of blood is as much as 9 times that of water.

The physiologic unit for resistance to flow is the peripheral resistance unit (PRU). It is defined as the pressure gradient in mm. Hg divided by the flow in ml. per second. It comes as no surprise that when the average circulatory flow of 100 ml. per sec. is divided into the average circulatory pressure gradient from artery to vein of 100 mm. Hg, the normal PRU obtained equals 1.

$$PRU = \frac{100 \text{ mm. Hg}}{100 \text{ ml./sec.}} = 1$$

Typical PRU's for various conditions are listed in Table 4.4.

Blood pressure tends to reduce vascular resistance, since it holds open the vessels against the vasomotor tone of the external muscles. As the pressure drops, there is a point at which the external collapsing force is no longer opposed and the vessel closes. This is especially

---

* Hematocrit is determined by centrifuging coagulated blood for 30 minutes at 1500 ft. per sec.², after which the ratio of red cell volume to total volume constitutes the measurement.

true for the arterioles, which are the valves of the circulatory system. The critical closing pressure for a normal arteriole is 20 mm. Hg. However, if the sympathetic division of the ANS inhibits the muscle, the arteriole will not close until a pressure of 0 mm. Hg is reached. If the sympathetic division of the ANS stimulates the muscle, the vessel may close at a pressure of 60 mm. Hg. Consequently, the vessel will be nearly closed all the time—an indication of the constrictor effect of sympathetic innervation.

Capacitance has been defined as the change in volume produced by a unit change in pressure. The physiologist defines vascular compliance (VC) as the total volume of blood that can be stored for each mm. Hg increase in pressure. Vascular compliance is the capacitance of the vascular vessel. Vascular distensibility (VD) is defined as the fraction increase in volume for each mm. Hg rise in pressure.

$$VC = \Delta Q/P$$

$$VD = \frac{\Delta Q}{\text{vol.}} \cdot \frac{1}{P}$$

Hence,

$$VC = VD \times \text{vol.}$$

Where VC = vascular compliance
VD = vascular distensibility
Vol. = total volume of the vessel
ΔQ = change in volume of the blood in the vessel
P = blood pressure in mm. Hg

Vascular compliance is vascular distensibility times volume.

The vascular distensibility for each vessel can be measured. Thus, the venous system is six times as distensible as the arterial system, and has four times its volume. This means that the capacitance of the venous system is $6 \times 4 = 24$ times that of the arterial system. When a sudden threat causes the heart to beat more rapidly, it increases the blood pressure of the arteries and decreases the pressure in the veins. But the effect on the arterial system is 24 times as great as the effect on the veins.

In the reverse direction, when an accident causes a hemorrhage, the blood pressure in the artery drops, but the veins constrict, providing additional circulation and maintaining the system for a loss of blood of as much as 25% of the total volume of the system.

Fluid flow through living tissues follows the principles of fluid dynamics. Hemodynamics is a division of fluid dynamics until extraordinary conditions occur, such as when the arterioles constrict until their bore approaches the diameter of a red blood cell, at which time the red blood cell blocks the flow completely. Normally, streamline flow occurs in most blood vessels. But at the opening of the heart valves turbulent flow occurs for a short time, producing sounds which the physician can detect with the stethoscope (Korotkoff's sounds).

CONTROL OF BLOOD PRESSURE

Having defined the parameters of our system (R, C, I, and E), we now need to see how the body employs control techniques to supply adequate blood flow to each organ, and yet maintains the systemic blood pressure within close tolerances. As in all of nature's control mechanisms, redundancy is prominent. Three methods are employed: nervous regulation of blood pressure, kidney regulation of blood pressure, and control of blood pressure by the endocrine glands.

The nervous regulation of blood pressure is performed by the sympathetic division of the ANS Pressure receptors in the aorta and carotid arteries have a nonlinear response curve, which possesses maximum response at the normal level of blood pressure. Hence, a small increase in blood pressure causes a large increase in signal, triggering the vasomotor control center in the lower pons and upper medulla of the brainstem. The vasomotor center keeps the vasoconstrictor fibers in the blood vessels tonically active at all times.

When a high blood pressure signal comes from the receptors, the action of the vasomotor center is inhibited, causing vasodilatation in the peripheral circulatory system, and a decrease in cardiac rate and force. The blood pressure drops, the pressure receptors lose their inhibitory effect on the vasomotor center, muscle tone in the blood vessels increases, and pressure rises. This control loop is used to control blood pressure during rapid stresses, e.g., changes in posture, bleeding, and exercise. The long-term regulation of blood pressure is produced by the kidney controls and by the endocrine glands.

The control mechanism exercised by the kidney can be verified by placing a clamp so as to restrict the blood flow through the renal artery. During a period of weeks, the systemic blood pressure gradually increases until the kidney blood pressure returns to its former value. When the constriction is removed, the systemic blood pressure returns to that required to maintain proper renal artery pressure. The possible mechanism for renal control of arterial pressure may be summarized as follows:

1.) A drop in arterial pressure produces a drop in renal pressure, which in turn causes a drop in renal efficiency.

2.) Water and electrolytes are retained in blood.

3.) Aldosterone increases extracellular fluid volume, total blood volume, mean systemic pressure, heart rate and flow of blood through tissues.

4.) Tissues attempt to reduce flow by increasing resistance.

5.) Increased resistance leads to an increase in arterial pressure.

Three endocrine secretions can affect arterial pressure: vasopressin, norepinephrine, and aldosterone. Vasopressin, formed in the hypothalamus, is also called ADH (antidiuretic hormone) because it controls the absorption of water by the kidney. Norepinephrine and epinephrine are formed in the adrenal glands and circulate through the bloodstream. They stimulate the muscular tunics of the walls of the blood vessels in a manner similar to the sympathetic division of the ANS. They constitute a back-up support, but in times of emergency furnish a quick way to constrict the muscles to prevent loss of blood and maintain the blood pressure. Aldosterone, secreted by the adrenal cortex, has a major effect on extracellular fluid volume and sodium content. To exert its effect it enters the control loop at step 3 in the foregoing outline and controls the blood pressure by varying the fluid volume in the body.

THE CENTRAL PUMP

The heart as a pump contains four stages: two input stages and two output stages. The input stages are the atria. The right atrium admits the blood returned from the veins of the system. The left atrium admits the blood returned from the lungs. Each input stage is connected to its output stage by a valve—the mitral valve on the left and the tricuspid valve on the right. The force of cardiac contraction causes the opening of the atrial valves and forces the blood into the output stage, the ventricle. From the right ventricle the blood is pumped to the lungs; from the left ventricle the blood is pumped through the entire circulatory system. The blood passes from the left ventricle through the aortic valve into the aorta. Blood from the right ventricle proceeds through the pulmonary valve into the pulmonary artery. The contraction phase of the heart is called the systole; the relaxation phase, the diastole.

The heart is the source of all pressures in the body fluids. The fluid entering the right atrium is considered to be at zero pressure, i.e., at atmospheric pressure. (A mercury manometer connected at this point would not be lifted against the atmospheric pressure pushing down upon it.) The pressure of the blood emerging from the right ventricle is approximately 25 mm. Hg; from the left ventricle it is about 120 mm. Hg.

During the relaxation phase the left atrium is open to the fluid returning to it from the lungs; the right atrium is open to the fluid returning to it from the body. As the wall of the atrium contracts, very little increase in pressure results. The fluid is merely transferred to the ventricle. Within 0.2 seconds the ventricle contracts, closing the atrioventricular (A-V) valve, building up to 80% of its pressure before the exit valve opens. It continues to squeeze with the valve open, increasing the pressure to its maximum. The pressure then drops sufficiently to close the valve. Output pressure is maintained with the valve closed. The internal pressure in the ventricles drops as the heart muscle relaxes in its diastole. At the same time, the next cycle has started at the atrium, and approximately 0.8 seconds have elapsed; total systole = 0.27 seconds, total diastole = 0.53 seconds.

Observed from the mechanical pump that is the heart are certain sounds related to its operation. The physician hears them each time he places a stethoscope to a patient's chest. The sounds can be amplified with a microphone and loudspeaker. The phonocardiograph records the sounds by placing a recording galvanometer in the output of the audio amplifier.

The pumping action of the heart roughly approximates the sound *lub-dub, lub-dub,* indicating two sounds. When the pressure and the sound of the heart are recorded on the same chart, the first heart sound appears as the A-V valve closes, and continues until the aortic and pulmonary valves open. The second heart sound appears at the end of systole. It starts when the aortic and pulmonary valves open and stops when the A-V valve closes.

Additional sounds are recorded by the phonocardiogram. Heart sound 3 is heard while the ventricle is being filled. Heart sound 4 is the sound of blood being pushed from the atrium through the partially open A-V valve. This sound can be heard only in a defective heart in which ventricular contraction is absent.

Murmurs are produced by turbulent flow, usually of defective hearts. Sometimes during exercise, the blood moves rapidly enough to produce turbulence during normal heart cycles. Stenosis, or contraction of valve opening by scar tissue, causes heart murmur. Regurgitation, resulting from an improperly seated valve, causes murmur. Aortic stenosis is murmur during systole; mitral stenosis occurs during diastole. Aortic regurgitation occurs during diastole; mitral regurgitation occurs during systole.

ELECTRICAL SIGNALS FROM THE HEART

The heart, composed of interconnected muscle fibers, can be subdivided into two discrete functional bundles: the atrial bundle and the ventricular bundle. These are connected by the A-V bundle. Stimulation of any part of the atrial bundle causes the action potential to affect the entire atrium. Stimulation of any part of the ventricular bundle causes the action potential to engulf the entire ventricle. The A-V bundle carries the signal from atrium to ventricle and back. Note in Figure 4.4 that the action potential of the cardiac muscle has a plateau, which causes the action potential to last much longer in cardiac than in skeletal muscle. The muscle contraction period is close to the duration of the action potential, i.e., about 0.15 seconds in atrial muscle, and 0.3 seconds in ventricular muscle.

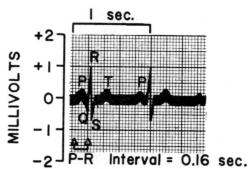

Figure 4.4 Standard electrocardiogram. (From A. C. Guyton *Textbook of Medical Physiology* (3d ed.). Philadelphia: Saunders, 1966.)

Just below the opening of the superior vena cava into the heart is a node of specialized muscle, the sinoatrial (S-A) node. This is the pacemaker of the heart. If left alone it will depolarize itself in a natural period of 70 to 80 beats per minute. The S-A fibers are continuous with the fibers of the atrium. The entire atrium is stimulated by the S-A node. The signal is conducted through the atrium until it reaches the A-V node where the signal is delayed about 0.1 second to allow the blood to enter the ventricles. Conduction to the fibers of the ventricle is by a bundle of conductive tissue called the Purkinje fibers, which produce almost immediate transmission. The signal spreads through the ventricle to complete the contraction in 0.2 seconds.

The electrocardiogram (ECG) is a recording of the electrical impulses originating in the heart. The chart lines of the ECG are standardized. The horizontal scale represents time in seconds, a heavy line every 0.20 seconds, five interdigitating light lines representing 0.04 seconds per line. The chart moves at 25 mm. per second, so that every line = 1 mm. The vertical scale is calibrated in millivolts, 0.1 millivolt per (millimeter) division, using a standard millivolt signal to set the sensitivity of the recorder at 1 mv. per cm.

The graph presented by the normal heart is a PQRST-complex (Fig. 4.4). The first peak on the ECG is the P-wave, which represents the electrical impulse in the atrium. It is normally upward, 0.2 to 0.3 mv., and a duration of 0.08 second. Next comes the QRS complex, of which Q is often not visible. Q is a drop of perhaps 1 division followed by a large R peak, then a drop to a very low S, and a recovery to the base line. The QRS duration is about the same as the P, i.e., 0.08 second, about 2.5 mv. maximum height. It represents depolarization of the ventricles. The repolarization of the ventricles appears as a T wave, a 0.3 mv. peak of duration 0.16 seconds.

The electrocardiogram (ECG) is obtained by placing electrodes at standard positions on the patient's body. The "limb electrodes" are connected by cuffs to the right arm (RA), left arm (LA), and left leg (LL). The three standard leads are then characterized as follows:

Lead I RA–, LA+ (right arm is negative electrode; left arm is positive)

Lead II RA–, LL+ (right arm, negative; left leg, positive)

Lead III LA–, LL+ (left arm, negative; left leg, positive)

For more detailed studies, electrodes are placed in standard positions on the chest. Each chest position is measured in turn against a reference formed by connecting the standard limb leads, RA, LA, and LL, each through a 5000-ohm resistor to the negative side of the electrocardiograph machine.

THE RESPIRATORY SYSTEM

The respiratory system consists of all components required to pass air into and out of the lungs, transfer needed molecules from the air into the blood, carry materials to the cells, transfer materials to and from the cells, carry out the utilization of oxygen in the cells and the production of carbon dioxide and other waste products, transfer the waste products back to the blood and then to the lungs, excrete the products into lung air, and finally discharge into the atmosphere. The components and functions just described are summarized as follows:

From the atmosphere to 1.) *lungs* (breathing) to 2.) *blood* (diffusion) to 3.) *capillaries* (fluid flow) to 4.) *intracellular fluid* (transport) to 5.) *cell* (membrane transfer) to 6.) *mitochondria* (cellular respiration) to 7.) *cell* (diffusion and membrane transfer) to 8.) *intracellular fluid* (transport) to 9.) *capillaries* (membrane transfer) to 10.) *blood* (fluid flow) to 11.) *lungs* (transport) to 12.) *alveoli* (breathing) and back to the atmosphere.

BREATHING

Atmospheric air contains 78% nitrogen, 21% oxygen, 1% argon, 0.03% carbon dioxide, and traces of hydrogen, helium, and neon. In addition, it contains water vapor, dependent on the relative humidity at a particular time and place. Relative humidity is not an absolute quantity, but is a function of the temperature of the air. At every temperature, air has a saturation value, the maximum amount of moisture it can contain in vapor form, without its precipitation as a liquid. Thus, at body temperature (37°C), the saturation vapor pressure of air is 47 mm. Hg.

According to Dalton's law, the total pressure of a mixture of gases is equal to the sum of the partial pressures of the gases present. At 100% relative humidity, the vapor pressure of water at 37°C is 47 mm. Hg. At 50% relative humidity, the vapor pressure of water at

37°C is $^{47}/_2 = 23.5$ mm. Hg. The per cent water in the lung air (saturated) would be $^{47}/_{760} = 6.2\%$ (since the total pressure is 760 mm. Hg). Upon exhalation the air will cool to an atmospheric temperature of perhaps 22°C whose saturation water vapor pressure is 19.8 mm. Hg; hence, some of the water vapor must condense. On a cold day you can see the water vapor condense in the form of "steam" in the exhaled breath. At normal temperatures the moisture has a chance to be diluted in the atmosphere before it condenses.

Thus, the simple process of breathing—transporting air from room temperature to the lung environment—changes its relative humidity. Inhaled air of 50% humidity with respect to 22°C room temperature will be 20% humidity with respect to body temperature.

Without moisture (water-free basis), the gases in atmospheric air would have the partial pressures shown in Table 4.5.

The body regions that produce this concentration change include the mouth and nose where the air is inhaled and conditioned, the pharynx, the larynx, the trachea, the bronchi, the bronchioles, and the alveoli. In the lung sacs the air is brought close enough to pulmonary capillaries for gaseous diffusion to occur.

The alveoli (little sacs) are connected through bronchioles to the major passageways (bronchi) which converge on the major pipe (trachea) leading to the lungs. The entire assembly is sealed in the thoracic cavity by the pleura, and has the characteristics of a balloon sealed in a jar with a flexible cap.

If pressure is exerted on the diaphragm the internal pressure will cause partial collapse of the balloon, forcing the air out (exhalation). Downward tugging on the diaphragm will cause external air to rush in, filling the balloon (inhalation). Sealing the bottom of the thoracic cavity is the diaphragm, a powerful musculature that performs this function. In addition, the balloon itself is attached to the ribs, which can be moved by intercostal muscles to enlarge or contract the cavity.

During inspiration, not only are the lungs filled by the contraction of the diaphragm, but the rib cage overstretches the lungs to form an

TABLE 4.5   PARTIAL PRESSURE OF AIR MIXTURES (DRY BASIS)

Gas	Atmospheric %	Atmospheric mm. Hg	Expired %	Expired mm. Hg	Alveolar %	Alveolar mm. Hg
Nitrogen *	79.02	600.00	79.2	602.0	80.4	609.4
Oxygen	20.94	159.67	16.3	124.0	14.0	107.3
Carbon Dioxide	0.04	0.33	4.5	34.0	5.6	43.3
		760.00		760.0		760.0

* Because of the method of analysis, the nitrogen percentage includes other inert gases such as argon, helium, and neon.

internal (negative) pressure of −4 mm. Hg. During expiration, the abdominal muscles move the diaphragm back, and the thoracic cage can apply pressures as high as 40 mm. Hg on the lung walls.

No attempt is made to use the total lung capacity of 6000 ml. Each breath (tidal volume) amounts to about $\frac{1}{10}$ of this volume, or 500 ml. When 500 ml. is inhaled, only about 350 ml. reach the alveoli. The other 150 ml. fill the dead space, the trachea, and the bronchi in which sites no exchange takes place. If the air from the dead space is analyzed, it will be seen to have about the same composition as atmospheric air. In applying a respirator to a patient, one must be aware of the dead space of the respirator. If the volume of the dead space is 500 ml., no fresh air will reach the lung sacs, and the patient will suffocate.

Vital capacity is the total amount of air that can be moved into or out of the lungs. In addition to the tidal volume it includes the inspiratory reserve volume and the expiratory reserve volume. The difference between the vital capacity and the total lung capacity is the residual volume. In the discussion of instrumentation to measure these factors (Chapter 8), the importance of motivation of the patient is stressed in order to obtain the maximum inspiratory and expiratory volumes.

DIFFUSION OF GASES THROUGH MEMBRANES

When inhaled air is finally brought into the alveoli, the proper selection of gases diffuses through the membrane of the sac into the blood. The driving force for diffusion of a gas through a membrane is partial pressure difference:

$$\text{diffusion rate}_A = \frac{P_2 - P_1}{R} = \frac{\text{driving force}}{\text{resistance}}$$

The rate of diffusion of component A through a membrane is proportional to the gradient in partial pressures of that component across the membrane divided by the resistance to diffusion. The conductance in the diffusion process is called the diffusivity, $D = 1/R$. Hence,

$$\frac{dC_A}{dt} = D_A(P_o - P_{in})$$

where C_A = concentration of A inside the membrane (which is proportional to the partial pressure of A inside the membrane)

D_A = unit diffusivity of A through the membrane, i.e.,

$$\frac{\text{gas taken in per minute}}{\text{per mm. difference in partial pressure}}$$

P_o = partial pressure outside the membrane in mm. Hg
P_{in} = partial pressure inside the membrane in mm. Hg

Note that the diffusion will be *in* if P_o is greater than P_{in}, and *out* if P_o is less than P_{in}.

Calculation of the partial pressures of carbon dioxide and oxygen in alveolar air and in pulmonary blood will provide a measure of the size of the driving force toward diffusion. The partial pressures in the various sites including the partial pressure of water vapor are given in Table 4.6.

The diffusion coefficient for carbon dioxide is 20 times what it is for oxygen. Hence, even though there is a small composition gradient, the carbon dioxide is transferred to the lung air.

In the tissues the opposite effect takes place. The partial pressure of carbon dioxide can be 40 to 120 mm. Hg, depending on the metabolic rate of the cell. The oxygen concentration in the interstitial fluid is about 40 mm. Hg, at the arterial end of the capillary it is 95 mm. Hg, and at the venous end it is 40 mm. Hg.

CELL RESPIRATION

Cell respiration is the utilization of oxygen and nutrients in the cell to generate energy and produce waste products, such as carbon dioxide. Earlier we had pointed out that this occurred in the mitochondria of the cell, and that the Krebs cycle was used to convert the oxygen and nutrients to ATP, the universal energy source. Figure 4.5 shows the chemical structure of ATP. Each one of the three phosphate groups liberates 7000 calories

$$\text{ATP} \xrightarrow{7000 \text{ cal.}} \text{ADP} \xrightarrow{7000 \text{ cal.}} \text{AMP}$$

ATP is formed by carbohydrate metabolism, essentially from the monosaccharide glucose. Glucose is converted first to pyruvic acid and then to acetyl-coenzyme. In the Krebs cycle the acetyl portion of this molecule is degraded to carbon dioxide and hydrogen, while the

TABLE 4.6 PARTIAL PRESSURE OF GASES IN PULMONARY SYSTEM

| Gas | Moist Basis, mm. Hg | | | Pulmonary Circulation | |
	Atmosphere	Alveolar Air	Expired Air	Arterial Blood	Venous Blood
Nitrogen	597.0	569	566	564	569
Oxygen	159.0	104	120	40	104
Carbon Dioxide	0.3	40	27	45	40
Water Vapor	3.7	47	47	47	47
	760.0	760	760	696	760

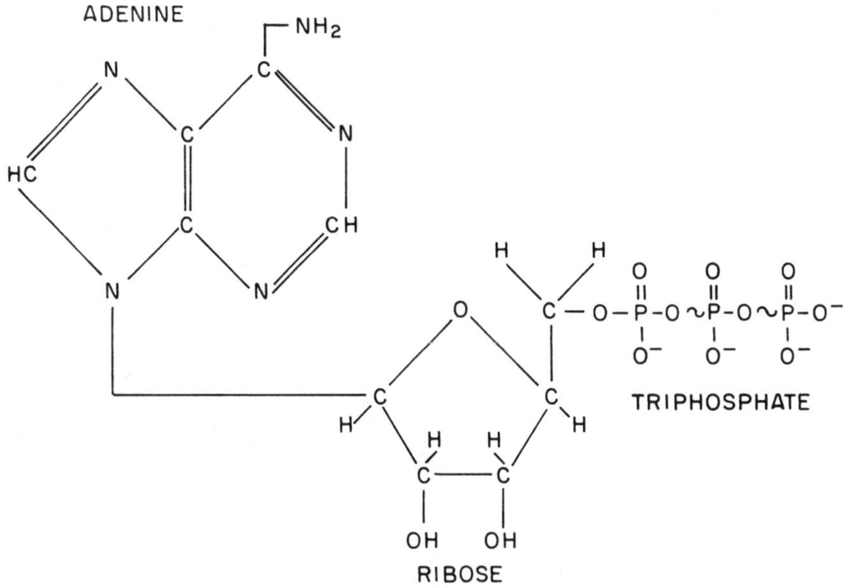

Figure 4.5 Chemical structure of adenosine triphosphate (ATP).

coenzyme portion is regenerated and ADP is converted to ATP. The overall reaction is

$$2 \text{ Acetyl Co-A} + 6H_2O + 2ADP \rightarrow 4CO_2 + 16H + 2 \text{ Co-A} + 2ATP$$

(Krebs cycle)

CONTROL OF RESPIRATION

The respiratory control center in the medulla and lower pons adjusts the respiration of the body to control the partial pressure of alveolar oxygen (P_{O_2}) and the partial pressure of alveolar carbon dioxide (P_{CO_2}). In the control center are found some neurons that discharge during inspiration and some that discharge during expiration.

Physiologists postulate that what we have here is a neuronal oscillator that inspires for 2 seconds and expires for 3 seconds. If one of the inspiration neurons becomes excited, the signal spreads to all of them. After all the neurons have repeatedly fired for 2 seconds, they become fatigued and the pulse stops. The expiratory neurons are also stimulated to fire, but during the inspiratory period they are inhibited by signals from the inspiratory neurons. When the inspiratory cycle is completed, however, the inhibitory signal disappears and the expiratory neurons can now fire. They continue to fire for about 3 seconds, when fatigue sets in. While expiration is taking place, the inspiratory neurons have recovered from their fatigue. They would fire except that they are restrained by the inhibitory signal emanating from the expiratory neurons. When the expiration cycle is completed, however, the inhibitory signal disappears and the inspiration can again start.

How is this oscillator principle overridden by higher control elements? The reflex described by Hering and Breuer in 1868 involves the stretch receptors in the lungs. As the lungs expand, the stretch receptors send impulses to the respiratory center through the vagus nerve to inhibit inspiration and to initiate expiration.

The pneumotaxic reflex comes from a center in the pons, which is stimulated by the inspiratory center to inhibit inspiration and initiate expiration. It is a timed reflex and apparently can speed up or slow down respiration when other centers of the brain require such action. Experimental evidence shows that respiration rate can be altered by 1.) the thought of doing exercise, 2.) impulses from muscles that they are being used (exercise), 3.) reduction in P_{O_2} of the blood, 4.) increase in P_{CO_2} of the blood, and 5.) change in pH of the blood.

In addition, there are chemoreceptors in the carotid and aortic bodies sensitive to oxygen, carbon dioxide, pH, and temperature, which furnish control when the primary control mechanisms fail — another of nature's fail-safe mechanisms which we have been observing in each physiologic control system.

RESPIRATORY MEASUREMENTS

This section deals with the conventional instruments for the measurement of respiratory variables. The new instrumental methods will be discussed in subsequent chapters.

The spirometer is the classic instrument for the measurement of pulmonary variables. It is simply a drum inverted in a cylinder of water. The drum is filled with air, and its position is recorded by a simple cord connection to a kymograph (a cylinder of paper rotated by a spring marked by a pen on an arm). As the patient breathes in and out, the volumes change the displacement of the drum, which when recorded can be used to calculate the required volumes from the calibration factor of the apparatus. Parameters like tidal volume, inspiratory reserve volume, and expiratory reserve volume can be recorded.

The spirometer filled with oxygen, and containing soda lime to remove the carbon dioxide formed, can be used as a metabolator to measure the basic metabolism of a patient. The oxygen consumed is given an energy equivalent of 4.825 calories per liter. This is the average energy liberated by the body per liter of oxygen.

The diffusivity of the respiratory membrane can be measured by measuring carbon monoxide diffusivity. A very small sample of carbon monoxide is breathed in, and the partial pressure of carbon monoxide is measured in subsequent air samples. Since the hemoglobin of the blood completely absorbs carbon monoxide, it is assumed that the P_{CO} of the blood is zero. Hence, the driving force is the P_{CO} in the alveolus itself. By measuring the amount of carbon monoxide absorbed in a given time and dividing it by the partial pressure, the diffusivity for carbon monoxide is obtained. The oxygen diffusivity is 1.23 times that of carbon monoxide. Typical test results show 17 ml. per minute diffusion for carbon monoxide and 21 ml. per minute for oxygen.

CONTROL OF BODY FLUIDS

One of the most significant gains that has been made in hospital care in the past 20 years is in the control of body fluids of sick or surgically incapacitated individuals. Seriously ill patients have difficulty in maintaining the proper balance between extracellular and intracellular fluids. The understanding of the control of this balance is one of the achievements of modern medicine that has reduced hospital mortality.

OSMOTIC CONTROL OF FLUIDS

Whenever a membrane separates two regions containing solutions of different concentration, the water will tend to move through the membrane to equalize the concentrations. If pressure is applied in the reverse direction to prevent the water from migrating, the amount of pressure required to prevent this movement is the *osmotic pressure* of the water at the other side of that membrane. Molecules of salt, electrolytes, or proteins reduce this osmotic pressure in proportion to their number. Hence, osmotic pressure is used by physical chemists to measure the number of molecules present. When a salt ionizes, each ion has the effect of a molecular particle in reducing osmotic pressure. Each ion in the body has its effect on the osmolality (osmotic pressure) of the solution in which it is found. If one adds up the osmolality of the materials in the three fluids of the body—plasma, extracellular, and intracellular fluid—they each equal a total osmotic pressure of 5340 mm. Hg. This means that if a cell is surrounded by pure water, the water would diffuse into the cell in an attempt to reduce the intracellular concentration with a force of about 7 atmospheres. The cell would explode.

Osmotic control of body fluids is performed by small changes in this large number. If water is removed from the body by perspiration, or by excessive urination, it diffuses from the extracellular area. This causes fluid to diffuse from the cells, producing dehydration. The function of these cells is impaired until water is returned. The body initiates its control mechanism to remedy this lack.

Normal Blood Volumes

The total amount of water in the standard (70 kg.) man is 40 liters. The water is distributed between the extracellular fluid (15 liters) and the intracellular fluid (25 liters). The blood volume of 5 liters consisting of 3 liters of plasma and 2 liters of fluid in the red cells is not included in this total.

Measurement of the body fluid volume can be performed by a dilution technique. A small quantity of dye or radioactive material is injected into the desired cavity. It is allowed to disperse until uniformly distributed throughout a body area. The volume of fluid in a body cavity is determined by dividing the total quantity of dye injected by the concentration measured in that cavity.

Concentration of dye per unit volume × volume of cavity = total amount of dye injected.

Thus,

$$\text{volume of cavity} = \frac{\text{total amount of dye injected}}{\text{concentration of dye measured}}$$

Blood volume is difficult to determine because a dye or radioactive material added to the blood diffuses rapidly into the extracellular volume and into the cells. A material that reacts with the protein in the blood plasma, or one that reacts with the blood cells, would remain permanently in the blood. Radioactive iron, chromium, or phosphate react with blood cells. Vital dyes and radioactive iodine will combine with plasma protein. For example, when Cr^{51} is used, a sample of blood is taken from the patient and incubated with the radioactive material until the reaction is complete. The total content of Cr^{51} is measured, the sample is injected into the patient, and the dilution method is carried out as with the dye in the extracellular fluid.

Extracellular fluid volume is measured by a material that will leave the blood and stay in the extracellular fluid. Radioactive sodium, chloride, bromide, and sucrose have been used. None of these substances gives reproducible results because they all diffuse into the cells in different amounts and at different rates. The practice is to define the fluid space in terms of the material used, calling it the "sodium space," the "sucrose space," and so forth. Inulin has been used in a somewhat different manner, based on the fact that it is rapidly and totally excreted in the urine. Inulin is injected slowly into the subject, and the concentration in the plasma is repeatedly measured until it becomes constant. The injection is then stopped, and the material is allowed to accumulate in the urine. The quantitative analysis of inulin in the urine is taken as the total inulin in the body. The extracellular fluid volume can be calculated from the following equation:

$$\text{volume of extracellular fluid} = \frac{\text{total inulin added}}{\text{constant concentration of inulin in plasma}}$$

FUNCTION OF THE CAPILLARIES

The 3.5 billion capillaries cover 4500 sq. cm. of area in carrying materials from the blood at low pressure to the cells of the body. The capillaries provide an interlocking circuit of many paths between the arteriole and the venule, and between the artery and the vein. At the proximal end of each capillary there is a sphincter which controls the flow through the capillary. This sphincter is either open or closed. The flow through each capillary of any area is either full or zero. The pulses are adjusted to maintain the required oxygen concentration in the adjacent tissue. As each pulsation moves fluid through a capillary, a large amount of dissolved particles and water molecules diffuse back and forth through the capillary wall, at least 40 times as rapidly as the plasma flows through the capillary.

Gases (oxygen and carbon dioxide) diffuse through the lipid walls of the capillaries. The electrolytes diffuse through pores. The plasma is mainly protein and cannot diffuse through either the capillary walls or the pores. Its large molecular weight inside the capillary tends to move fluid inward through the membrane by osmotic pressure. There are also colloids in the interstitial spaces which produce the opposite osmotic effect. The liquid pressure in the capillary is aided by a negative fluid pressure in the extracellular area. Values of fluid and osmotic pressures accepted by physiologists include the following:

Capillary fluid pressure (mm. Hg)
arterial end of capillary   40
venous end of capillary   20
average capillary pressure   30

Capillary osmotic pressure (mm. Hg)
arterial end of capillary   1
venous end of capillary   3

Interstitial fluid pressure   = 5 mm. Hg
Interstitial osmotic pressure = 26 mm. Hg

Table 4.7 summarizes the relationship between the osmotic and fluid pressures in the capillaries. At the arterial end a net pressure of 10 mm. Hg forces fluid out of the capillaries into the interstitial area. At the venous end of the capillaries a net pressure of 8 mm. Hg forces fluids from the interstitial area into the capillaries.

FUNCTIONS OF THE LYMPHATIC SYSTEM

The lymphatic system provides a route for fluids to return from the interstitial spaces to the blood. Proteins that may diffuse out of the capillaries cannot be returned by any other than the lymphatic route. The osmotic balance in the interstitial tissues requires careful control of the protein and fluid concentration.

TABLE 4.7 DRIVING FORCES IN CAPILLARY BEDS (all units in mm. Hg)

Arterial End		Venous End	
Internal Pressure		Internal Pressure	
fluid pressure	40	fluid pressure	20
osmotic pressure	1	osmotic pressure	3
Total internal	41 mm Out	Total internal	23 mm Out
External Pressure		External Pressure	
fluid pressure	5	fluid pressure	5
osmotic pressure	26	osmotic pressure	26
Total external	31 mm In	Total external	31 mm In
Net Pressure	10 mm Out	Net Pressure	8 mm In

The lymphatic system is a network of vessels, about the size of capillaries, which drain into larger vessels and ultimately empty into the veins. The lymphatic pressure is always lower than the tissue pressure, and hence any fluid accumulating in the tissues drains into the lymph glands. In addition to removal of fluid the lymphatic system contains lymph nodes which function to combat infection. Bacteria are detained at the nodes and antibodies are formed which go through the body. The lymph glands that pass through the abdominal area are responsible for the absorption of fats from the intestines.

Motion through the lymph glands is brought about by pressure from exercising muscles. Each time a muscle is used it squeezes the lymph gland near it. The lymphatics contain valves which allow motion in only one direction. Hence, flows of 100 ml. per hour to 1400 ml. per hour are found.

The accumulation of protein in the tissue builds up an osmotic pressure which *decreases* resorption of fluid and thus *increases* fluid. This increased fluid pressure increases the flow of the fluid and the protein into the lymphatic system. Without this continuous removal of protein and excess fluid, the functioning of the capillaries would be impaired.

HOW THE KIDNEY WORKS

The kidneys have two functions—to excrete waste and to control the chemical concentration of the materials in the body fluids. As we shall see, the functions are interrelated. The active element of the kidney is the nephron. A typical kidney has 1 million of these filtering systems to clean the blood plasma of unwanted substances.

In the nephron the blood to be purified passes through the glomerulus where about 1/5 of the plasma diffuses into Bowman's capsule (which surrounds the glomerulus). The filtered material passes through a tubule, a long loop of Henle, a distal tubule, and a collecting duct. While doing so, all the valuable materials are resorbed by the adjacent blood vessels. All the wastes leave the kidney through the collecting duct. About ⅕ of the total cardiac output of blood passes through the kidneys at any one time. This means that about 180 liters of fluid daily is resorbed in the capillaries of the kidneys.

The normal filtration pressure difference between the blood side and the kidney side is about 24 mm. Hg. The filtration rate is directly proportional to the pressure. When sympathetic stimulation requires reduction in blood flow to the kidney, both the afferent and efferent arterioles become constricted, reducing the blood flow but keeping the filtration pressure constant. When arterial pressure rises, the afferent arteriole closes, maintaining the pressure at the capsule and the filtration rate constant. When large quantities of water are consumed, the plasma protein is diluted, an action that reduces the inverse osmotic pressure and increases the filtration rate to remove the increased levels of water from the blood.

How does the tubule work? Like any other membrane it acts by both active and passive transport. Sodium is removed by active transport. Both an electrochemical gradient and a concentration gradient transport sodium from the blood to the cell of the tubule. But sodium exits from the cell against the electrochemical and concentration gradients, and this requires active transport of the kind that uses ATP, the sodium pump previously described. To remove water from the blood after the tubule cell has removed sodium ions, the peritubular fluid has a higher concentration of solute than the blood fluid, and water diffuses out by osmosis. Negative ions like chloride, phosphate, and bicarbonate are attracted by the positive charge of the sodium ions in the tubules and diffuse across under electrical gradients. After the water is absorbed, the blood urea concentration increases and is absorbed by a concentration gradient. Later, in the tubule system when resorption takes place, the membrane limits resorption of certain molecules like urea, creatinine, inulin, mannitol, and sucrose. Once these materials enter the filtrate, they stay there until discharged in the urine.

The membrane of the nephron is different at each location in the kidney. At the first location—the proximal tubule—all the glucose, amino acids, and proteins as well as 80% of the water, sodium, potassium, and chloride are reabsorbed. The cells of the proximal tubules are large and contain large numbers of mitochondria to supply the ATP needed for active transport. The loop of Henle which is the structure next in the filtration train has a highly permeable descending side, but the ascending side is impermeable to water and absorbs sodium and chloride rapidly. In the distal tubules urine is finally prepared. Here the permeability to water can be controlled by anti-diuretic hormone (ADH). In the absence of this hormone the membrane is almost impermeable to water.

In the distal tubules, a procedure is available for the concentration of the urine, if the body is suffering from a water shortage. The active transport of sodium that occurred earlier increases the osmotic gradient for water in the distal convoluted tubule. Water is resorbed in a special vessel where the blood is moving slowly, and the high solute concentration absorbs a great volume of water. Hence, when the command is given from the adenohypophysis, the kidneys can control the loss of water from the body.

CONTROL OF CHEMICAL COMPOSITION

The concentration of electrolytes in the fluids surrounding the cells must remain within very narrow limits in order for the cells to operate efficiently. Sodium, potassium, calcium, and magnesium (cations) and chloride, bicarbonate, and phosphate (anions) are all controlled by kidney function. Just as we saw that ADH can control the elimination of water at a normal rate of 15 to 18 ml. per minute to a rate as low as 0.35 ml. per minute, other hormones can control the resorption rate of electrolytes by the collecting duct.

The control system employed by aldosterone to regulate the concentration of sodium in the body is a *biochemical reflex*. A 5% decrease in sodium concentration will increase the production of aldosterone by the adrenal cortex, which in turn increases the absorption of sodium in the distal collecting tubules. When potassium concentration increases by 25%, the aldosterone rate is increased, reducing the resorption of potassium. The mechanism is apparently an ion-exchange type, sodium ions being resorbed and potassium ion being secreted. Thus, the sodium to potassium ratio is also regulated.

Calcium is a very valuable ion because it is required for muscular contraction; a low calcium level in extracellular fluid will disturb the musculature of the heart. When calcium concentration drops, the secretion of parathyroid hormone is stimulated, which increases calcium resorption in the renal tubules.

Negative ions such as chloride and bicarbonate are affected because of their relation to the transfer of ions like sodium and potassium. Thus when aldosterone promotes increased sodium transfer, the negative chloride ions are also transferred to obtain electrical neutrality.

Similarly, parathyroid hormone controls phosphate by allowing more of it to be excreted in the kidney, while it is also increasing calcium resorption.

THE FLUID CONTROL SYSTEM

There are two fluid control systems operating in the body including 1) the day-to-day servosystem which adjusts rate of fluid removal to match the rate of fluid intake; and 2) the emergency system in which hormones are released by the hypophysis upon command of the osmoreceptor that the osmotic pressure in the blood has dropped too low. Block diagrams of both systems are shown in Figure 4.6.

The fluid-balancing mechanism that operates continually uses the glomerular filtration rate of the kidney to control fluid removal from the body. If intake exceeds removal, fluid will accumulate in the tissues and in the blood. This increase of fluid in the tissues will promote increased tissue pressure and increased diffusion of fluids into the blood, producing increased blood pressure in capillaries, veins, and finally arteries. Increased arterial pressure will cause more diffusion of fluids at the renal nephron and thus increase water removal.

Hormonal Fluid Control Mechanism

Body fluid is controlled by a balance between the fluid intake and the fluid excretion. The osmotic pressure of the blood is sensitive to

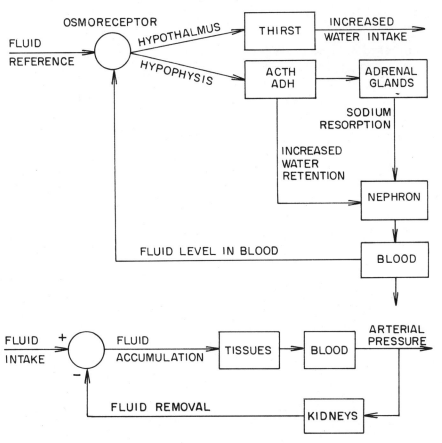

Figure 4.6 Fluid control mechanism. *A*, Hormonal control (emergency system); *B*; Fluid-balancing mechanism (servosystem).

the total fluid concentration in the body. Osmoreceptors in the hypothalamus respond to the osmotic pressure of the blood, and the hypothalamus reacts by producing a sensation of thirst. When an animal responds to the thirst signal, he drinks only enough water to restore osmotic balance to the blood. The osmoreceptor does not detect the change until a later time when the water has been absorbed and enters the circulatory system.

A second signal from the osmoreceptors activates the hypophysis (pituitary gland) to produce more antidiuretic hormone (ADH), which affects the resorption of water in the tubules of the kidneys. Hence, the osmoreceptors stimulate both the imbibing of more and the excretion of less water.

The osmoreceptors also stimulate the hypophysis to secrete ACTH (adrenocorticotropic hormone), which stimulates the cortex of the adrenal glands to produce aldosterone. This hormone affects the sodium resorption in the kidney, which also stimulates additional water resorption. It then acts to preserve both the sodium and the water content of the body. (See Fig. 4.6.)

Control of Acid-Base Balance

The acid-base balance of the body is carefully controlled so that the pH * of the arterial blood is always precisely 7.41. Venous blood pH will vary with the carbon dioxide being removed from the body to levels averaging 7.36. The intercellular fluid pH will also vary with the metabolism of the local cells from 6.0 to 8.5. Control of the acid-base balance in the body is effected primarily by the *buffer* system, which will be explained shortly. Other measures that support this system include increased respiration to remove excess carbon dioxide from the blood, and secretion of acid or alkaline urine by the kidneys for long-range equalization. These effects are direct and rapid. Thus, when the pH changes, the respiratory control center increases respiration almost immediately to get rid of excess carbon dioxide and increase the pH. The kidney acts automatically, by responding to the chemical change in body fluids to discharge more acidic urine when the pH is low and more alkaline urine when the pH is high.

Buffering action is produced when a weak acid, a weak base, or a salt is present in a solution. The ionization of acetic acid, for example, can be represented by

$$\text{HAc} \rightleftharpoons \text{H}^+ + \text{Ac}^-$$

and the ionization constant formula:

$$\frac{[\text{H}^+][\text{Ac}^-]}{(\text{HAc})} = \text{K}_{\text{ion}} = 1.00 \times 10^{-5}$$

---

* Some of the information to be given in Chapter 5 about pH is vital at this point and should be consulted by the student. pH is the negative logarithm of the hydrogen ion concentration. The symbol "concentration of" is signified by placing brackets around the symbol for an ion, e.g., [Na$^+$] means the concentration of sodium ion.

If 0.1 molar acetic acid is used:

$$[HAc] = 0.1$$

and since from the above reaction $[H^+] = [Ac^-]$

$$[H^+][H^+] = [0.1][1 \times 10^{-5}] = 10^{-6}$$

$$[H^+] = 10^{-3}$$

$$pH = 3.00$$

If a sufficient amount of sodium acetate is added to the solution to make it 1.00 molar in acetate ion, the solution will be buffered because

$$[H^+][1.00] = [0.1][1 \times 10^{-5}]$$

$$[H^+] = 1 \times 10^{-6}$$

$$pH = 6.00$$

If 1 ml. of 10 N HCl is added to 1 liter of this solution, the additional hydrogen ion added will combine with some of the acetate to form acetic acid

$$[Ac^-] = {}^{10}\!/_{1000} \text{ less than before}$$

or

$$[H^+][Ac^-] = [H^+][1.00 - 0.01] = 1 \times 10^{-5}$$

$$[H^+] = 1.11 \times 10^{-6}$$

$$pH = -\log(1.11) + 6.00$$

$$pH = 5.95$$

If 1 ml. of 10 N NaOH were added to one liter of the original buffered solution, the OH$^-$ ions of the NaOH would react with the acetic acid

$$OH^- + HAc \rightarrow HOH + Ac^-$$

reducing the acetic acid concentration by the concentration of hydroxyl ion and increasing the acetate concentration by the same amount. The equation is

$$[H^+][1.00 + 0.01] = [0.100 - 0.01][1.00 \times 10^{-5}]$$

$$[H^+] = 8.91 \times 10^{-7}$$

$$pH = -\log(8.91) + 7.00 = 6.05$$

The effect of strong acid is to reduce the pH by 0.05; the effect of strong base increases the pH by 0.05. Without the buffer, the pH of the HCl added to the HAc would result mainly from the H$^+$ from the HCl

$$H^+ \text{ from } HAc = 1 \times 10^{-3}$$

$$H^+ \text{ from } HCl = 0.01 = 10^{-2}$$

$$\text{Total } [H^+] = 0.011 = 1.1 \times 10^{-2}$$

$$pH = 2.00 - \log 1.1 = 1.96$$

The pH of the NaOH would be mainly from the hydroxyl ion whose concentration $[OH^-] = 0.01$ since

$$[H^+][OH^-] = K_{H_2O} = 10^{-14}$$

$$[H^+][0.01] = 10^{-14}$$

$$[H^+] = 10^{-12}$$

$$pH = -\log (10^{-12}) = 12.00$$

Thus, without buffer, the pH can vary from 1.96 to 12.00. With buffer, the pH can vary from 5.95 to 6.05.

There are three buffer systems in the body:

1. The *bicarbonate buffer system* based on the weak acid, carbonic acid

$$H_2CO_3 \rightleftharpoons H^+ + HCO_3^-$$

which can also be written,

$$H_2O + CO_2 \rightleftharpoons H^+ + HCO_3^-$$

in the first form,

$$K = \frac{[H^+][HCO_3^-]}{[H^+]}$$

$$[H^+] = K \frac{[CO_2]}{[HCO_3^-]}$$

$$-\log H^+ = -\log K + \log \frac{[HCO_3^-]}{[CO_2]}$$

$$pH = pK + pCO_2 + \log[HCO_3^-], \text{ and the } pK = 6.1$$

The carbonate system is used by the kidneys to correct for large errors in the acid-base balance of the body.

2. The *phosphate buffer system* is based on NaH_2PO_4 and Na_2HPO_4

with a pK of 6.8

3. The *protein buffer system* based on the acid and basic radicals found in all amino acids (—COOH and NH_3OH) has an average pK of 7.4.

It is the major buffering system of the body, the protein in the system tending to buffer itself at a pH of 7.4.

SUMMARY

Physiology, as a branch of cybernetics, is concerned with the functioning of living systems. The cell itself, the basic element of an organic system, has been shown to contain subsystems, e.g., the mitochondria (the source of cell energy) and the endoplasmic reticulum (the cell chemical factory). Nerve cells have the ability to detect and transmit signals based on an electrochemical mechanism. Muscle cells have the ability to contract in response to nerve signals. Continuous signals can produce continuous contraction in the skeletal muscles. Cardiac muscle has a long refractory period; hence, it will contract and relax before it can contract again. Smooth muscle response is intermediate between that of cardiac and skeletal muscle.

The nervous system is the communication link in the feedback control systems of the body. The autonomic nervous system, by a combination of sympathetic and parasympathetic action, operates most of the principal organs of the body. The brain can override autonomic signals to a limited extent and can increase functions but cannot stop functions completely. Brain waves are signals of activity in the cortex of the brain, useful in diagnosing certain diseases. Biological transducers transmit mechanical, thermal, chemical, and electromagnetic information to the brain.

The circulatory system operates on the principles of flow through elastic carriers, and diffusion through membranes. Control of arterial pressure by the control of fluid volume is one of the functions of the kidneys. The endocrine glands provide an additional control system which takes over when the major system has allowed too much deviation, or in case of an emergency. The heart maintains the pressure and flow characteristics of the circulatory system. Its cycling can be monitored by its electrical and audio signals.

The respiratory system brings oxygen to the cells and removes carbon dioxide. Respiration includes the processes of breathing, diffusion of gases, flow of the fluids, mechanisms of membrane transport, and cell respiration.

The control of body fluids in the hospitalized patient is one of the gains that has made modern medicine so successful. Control is achieved by diffusion from the interstitial areas of the body to the capillaries or to the cells. The lymphatic system maintains the correct amount of plasma in the interstitial areas to provide the osmotic driving force required for proper fluid balance. The kidneys maintain fluid balance in the entire system by removing the amount of moisture required for the body conditions. The kidneys follow a servocontrol mechanism, driven by the total fluid level in the system. The nephron is the element in the kidney that removes wastes and controls fluid and electrolyte balance. The way in which it does this—by utilizing the principles of active transport, passive fluid transport, and osmotic transport—is a fascinating story.

EXERCISES

1. Use the known concentrations of sodium and potassium in the cell and in the surrounding fluid to calculate the Nernst potential of the resting cell. Explain your answer.

2. Look up the amino acids that occur in DNA and draw a part of the molecule.

3. Draw a block diagram for the control of the moisture level in the body by the kidneys.

4. Look up the details of the phosphate buffer system in a chemistry text and estimate the pH at which it buffers.

5 Look up the Krebs cycle in a medical physiology or biochemistry text and draw a block diagram of how it uses oxygen and glucose to make ATP from ADP.

6. Draw an ECG of a normal heart, and designate where the four heart sounds would appear. Show where mitral stenosis and mitral regurgitation murmurs would appear. Label the systolic and diastolic periods.

7. Draw canonical block diagrams for On-Off control, Servocontrol, and Regulator control and give two examples of where each is used in biological systems.

8. Show all the points at which analogies of Ohm's law have been used in the systems of the body.

9. Tabulate resistance and capacitance and list under each the analogous variable for blood flow, respiration, and membrane diffusion.

10. What are the most important instruments that need to be developed for the measurement of physiologic variables?

General Literature Cited and References

Crouch, J. E., and McClintic, J. R. Human Anatomy and Physiology. New York: Wiley, 1971.
Guyton, A. C. Textbook of Medical Physiology (3d ed.). Philadelphia: Saunders, 1966.
Langley, L. L. Outline of Physiology. New York: McGraw-Hill, 1961.
Ruch, T. C., and Patton, H. D. Physiology and Biophysics (19th ed.). Philadelphia: Saunders, 1965.
Taber, C. W. Cyclopedic Medical Dictionary (10th ed.). Philadelphia: Davis, 1965.

Chapter 5

Electrochemistry in Measurements

IN THE CELL, interstitial fluid, blood, and lymph, living tissue consists of fluids containing ions in solution. It is the controlled transfer of the ions in solution between these tissues that maintains life. Thus, the electrochemistry of these ions in solution is very important to the understanding, measurement, and control of the vital processes.

Electrochemistry dates from 1779 when Alessandro Volta stimulated frogs' legs by a voltage generated when dissimilar electrodes were placed into solutions containing ions. Quantitative electrochemistry dates from 1887 when Arrhenius formulated an ionic theory based on his measurements of ionic conductance, and from 1870 when Kohlrausch developed an improved resistance bridge. In 1909, Ostwald proposed the osmotic theory that we discussed in Chapter 4, and Debye improved on the theory of ions in solution and obtained the Nobel prize in 1936.

But electrochemistry which dates from the 18th century has only recently been useful in the hospital and clinic. It is the modern electronic revolution, with solid-state components providing stability of circuits, and short insulated leads preventing interference and pickup of extraneous signals that has made electrochemistry useful to the clinical technician and the laboratory physiologist.

Electrochemistry when properly applied can provide the dreamed-of transducer or the electrode which when inserted into a fluid indicates its composition, or which when inserted into the blood of a sick person provides data on pH, P_{CO_2}, and P_{O_2}. Without proper knowledge

113

and proper instrumentation, however, none of these determinations is possible.

Our topics from electrochemistry will include equilibrium of ions in solution, measurement of potential, current, conductivity, polarography, and selective ion electrodes.

EQUILIBRIUM OF IONS IN SOLUTION

An electrolyte is a substance which conducts electricity in solution by the transfer of ions. In order to do this, however, the electrolyte must separate into its constituent ions when dissolved in an appropriate solvent. The common electrolytes are acids, bases, and salts. Colloidal electrolytes consist of long hydrocarbon chains with an ionizable group at the end. Amino acids are colloidal electrolytes. Conduction through electrolytes is entirely different from that through ordinary conductors.

Metal conductors consist of fixed positively charged ions and a cloud of free electrons which conducts the current (and obeys Ohm's law). Electrolytic conductors contain both positive and negative ions. When a current is passed through the solution, the positive ions move toward the negative electrode and are called cations, and the negative ions move toward the positive electrode and are called anions. The negative ions move through a cloud of ions of opposite charge, as do the positive ions. The result is the theory of Debye and Huckel, as modified recently by Onsager and Fuoss.

The conductance of a solution at infinite dilution, when these effects are not present, and at finite dilution when the effects of the viscosity of the solution and the ionic cloud are felt, explains the deviation from theory of measured electrical conductances. For best theoretical effect, measurements should be made with no current flow; this is done in potentiometry, in which area differences between theory and measured potentials are due to contact potentials and to the overvoltage required to make the potential measurement. Devices must be developed and techniques used that compensate for these nonmeasurable quantities; these have been used in the form of reference electrodes and meters which are calibrated by using solutions of known potential, e.g., buffer solutions in pH measurements.

BASIC RULES

When an electrolyte is dissolved in water it dissociates to some extent into its ions, and an equilibrium is established that satisfies three rules.

The Conservation of Mass

The sum of the masses of the dissociated and undissociated parts is equal to the original mass. Thus, if acetic acid (HAc) is added to water, it dissociates only partially:

$$HAc \rightleftharpoons H^+ + Ac^-$$

But if 1 gram of acid is added to the solution, the sum of the weights of the ions from the acetic acid, the acetate ions, and the undissociated acetic acid will equal 1 gram.

The mass balance produces complications when a reaction takes place with the solvent. Thus, if 1 gram of sodium acetate is added to the solution, the salt will dissociate completely into 0.33 grams of sodium ion and 0.66 grams of acetate ion. But the acetate ion will react with the water to form 0.67 grams of acetic acid.

Electroneutrality

The sum of the negative ions will equal the sum of the positive ions. Thus, sodium bicarbonate dissociates in aqueous solution as follows:

$$NaHCO_3 \rightleftharpoons Na^+ + HCO_3^-$$

$$HCO_3^- \rightleftharpoons H^+ + CO_3^=$$

To achieve electroneutrality, the degree to which these reactions occur is such that the sum of the positive ions $Na^+ + H^+$ equals the sum of the negative ions $HCO_3^- + 2CO_3^=$.

Equilibrium Constants

The Law of Guldberg and Waage states that the rate of a chemical reaction is proportional to the concentrations of the reacting substances present at any time.

Thus, the rate at which H^+ reacts with Ac^- to form HAc is directly proportional to the $[H^+]$ * and $[Ac^-]$. Since, however, the HAc is decomposing at a rate proportional to its concentration, the reaction rates can be shown as follows:

1. $$r_1 = k_1[H^+][Ac^-] \quad \text{forward rate}$$

and

2. $$r_2 = k_2[HAc] \quad \text{reverse rate}$$

At equilibrium, the forward rate = the reverse rate, or

3. $$r_1 = r_2$$

4. $$k_1[H^+][Ac^-] = k_2[HAc]$$

5. $$K = \frac{k_1}{k_2} = \frac{[HAc]}{[H^+][Ac^-]}$$

---

* The symbol [] means "concentration of."

where K is the equilibrium constant of the reaction and is defined with the concentration of the products being in the numerator and the concentration of the reactants being in the denominator.

The Law of Guldberg and Waage applies to the "active concentrations" of ions, which for solids and pure liquids is considered constant.

SOLUBILITY PRODUCT

When a compound is only slightly soluble in water, its dissociation constant can be used to determine its solubility product. Thus, for calcium sulfate:

6. $$Ca^{++} + SO_4^= \rightleftharpoons CaSO_4 \text{ (slightly soluble)}$$

7. $$K_c = \frac{[CaSO_4]}{[Ca^{++}][SO_4^=]}$$

With the $[CaSO_4]$ considered a constant,

8. $$[Ca^{++}][SO_4^=] = [CaSO_4]/K_c = K_{SP}$$

K_{SP} is a constant, called the solubility product of $CaSO_4$. By the law of electroneutrality, $[Ca^{++}]$ equals $[SO_4^=]$. Hence, if by titration one could measure the $[Ca^{++}]$, one would find that

9. $$K_{SP} = [Ca^{++}]^2 = 6.1 \times 10^{-5}$$

$$= \text{the solubility product of this insoluble salt.}$$

IONIZATION CONSTANT

In a similar manner one can obtain the dissociation constant for weak acids and bases, which do not ionize completely. The ionization constant for acetic acid is defined as

$$K_i = \frac{[H^+][Ac^-]}{[HAc]}$$

and has an experimental value of 1.75×10^{-5}.

ION PRODUCT OF WATER

Another useful equilibrium constant is the ion product for water

$$K_{HOH} = [H^+][OH^-] = 10^{-14}$$

Hence, for absolute neutrality

$$[H^+] = [OH^-] = 10^{-7}$$

When a solution is acid, the hydrogen ion must be greater in concentration than 10^{-7}, and when a solution is basic, the $[H^+]$ must be less than 10^{-7}.

The pH is defined as $-\log[H^+]$, and it is less than 7 for an acid solution and greater than 7 for a basic solution.

ACTIVITY COEFFICIENT

All the principles of electrochemistry already outlined hold only at infinite dilution, i.e., when there is no attraction between the ions. At finite concentrations the solution properties hold for the *activity* of an ion, which is the concentration of the ion times its fugacity (freedom of motion), or the activity $(a_{ion}) = f_{ion} \times$ (conc. of ion).

We shall ignore this second order effect since most biological systems are dilute enough for the activity to be essentially equal to the concentration, i.e., the fugacity is essentially equal to one. However, when values are taken from tables, one should be certain that the activity at which the table was prepared is essentially equal to the activity at which the test is being made.

POTENTIOMETRIC MEASUREMENTS

Measurement of the electromotive force (e.m.f.) of galvanic cells is one of the most useful methods for studying the properties of electrolytes and the activity of ions in the body fluids. The e.m.f. measured in a galvanic cell, i.e., the voltage that appears on the meter (or other measuring system) contains two electrode potentials plus the two interface effects at the two electrodes (Fig. 5.1). The potential dif-

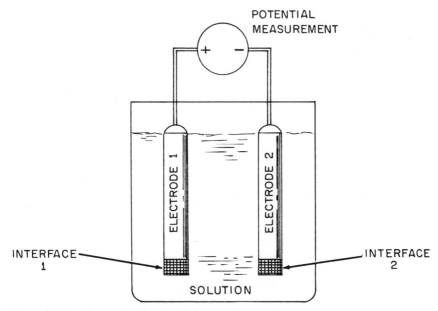

Figure 5.1 Elements of potential measurement.

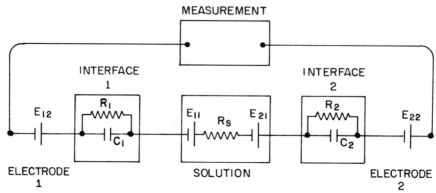

Figure 5.2 Electrical schematic of potential in solution.

ference between the electrodes is the galvanic potential, the interface effect at each electrode is the faradaic impedance (Fig. 5.2).

The electrochemical process at an electrode involves a transfer of charge from the solid phase of the electrode to the liquid phase of the solution, or vice versa. The interface effect at each electrode is a resistance-capacitance (RC) network which affects the dynamics and the rate of response, but not the steady-state potential, i.e., the potential with no current flow. What we really want to measure is the sum of the potentials generated at the four batteries shown in Figure 5.2, which are dependent on the chemical potentials of the ions and electrodes participating in the process. This quantity is called the e.m.f. of the electrode process (E). The e.m.f. at standard conditions (1 atm pressure and 25°C and all ions in solution at 1 M) is represented by E_o.

POTENTIOMETRY

Potentiometry is the measurement of the oxidation-reduction potential of a process, oxidation being defined as a loss of electrons (gain in positive charge), and reduction being defined as a gain of electrons (loss in positive charge). Hence, potentiometry is the measurement of the tendency of a system to gain or lose electrons; it is a measure of the e.m.f. available to move electrons, if a current of electrons were permitted to flow. In electrical terms it is the measure of the open circuit potential of the system.

It is convenient to separate a process into two half-cells—one (oxidation) where the solution loses electrons (the wire gains them), and the other (reduction) where the solution gains electrons (the wire loses them).

ELECTROCHEMICAL CELLS

An electrochemical cell can be prepared, consisting of a piece of zinc metal in a 1.0 M solution of Zn^{++}, a second half-cell is prepared, containing a piece of pure copper in a 1.0 M solution of Cu^{++}. Both half-cells are connected by a salt bridge. The electrochemist's notation for this system is

$$Zn/Zn^{++}//Cu^{++}/Cu$$

and the physical configuration appears in Figure 5.3.

The salt bridge provides liquid contact between the ions. Thus, if $ZnCl_2$ is dissolved in the Zn cell, and $CuCl_2$ is dissolved in the Cu cell, the salt bridge contains a KCl solution, held in place by an agar gel. Ions can diffuse through the salt bridge but no liquid will flow across. If the system is at standard conditions, we could look up the standard electrode potentials for Zn and Cu in a chemistry handbook and find that

$$Zn^{++} + 2e^- = Zn \quad -0.76 \text{ volts}$$

$$Cu^{++} + 2e^- = Cu \quad 0.34 \text{ volts}$$

The negative sign on the zinc equation means that the zinc will go into solution, giving off two electrons (oxidation), while the copper will be forced out of solution, absorbing the two electrons (reduction). The potential will be the sum of the two voltages: $0.76 + 0.34 = 1.10$ volts. By convention, for the electrochemical notation, the oxidation will be at the left, the reduction at the right, and the process moves from left to right. The cell would be symbolized by $\overline{Zn}/\overline{Zn}^{++}//Cu^{++}/Cu$.

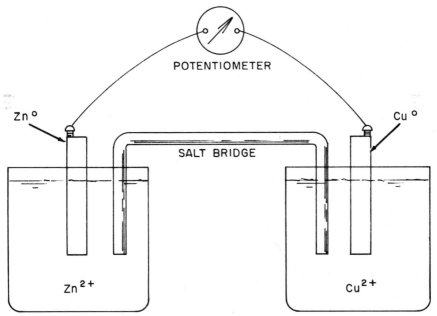

Figure 5.3 Physical configuration of potential measurement.

The overall chemical reaction that takes place is $Zn + Cu^{++} = Cu + Zn^{++}$. Indeed, if a piece of zinc metal is placed into a solution containing copper ions, the zinc goes into solution and the copper is plated out. By separating the reaction into two half-cells, we are able to measure the potential produced by this source.

STANDARD ELECTRODE POTENTIAL

Among the various ways of listing half-cell potentials, the Stockholm convention has been most widely accepted. This potential is obtained when the standard hydrogen electrode (SHE) is connected to the left of the electrode the standard potential of which is to be measured. As already indicated, the SHE is placed in the oxidizing position. Hence, when materials which reduce hydrogen from solution (metals above hydrogen in the electrochemical series) are tested, a negative potential is obtained. Based on the convention, materials above hydrogen in the electrochemical series have a negative standard potential, and materials below hydrogen in the series have a positive standard potential. The electrode configuration for establishing the standard electrode potential for zinc is $H_2(1 \text{ atm}),Pt/H^+(1 \text{ M})// Zn^{++}/Zn$. The physical configuration is shown in Figure 5.4. The potential measured is $E_0 = -0.763$.

If the same configuration is used for copper metal in contact with 1 M cupric chloride, a potential of $E_0 = 0.337$ is obtained. This means

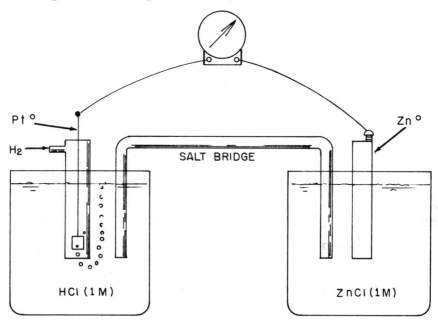

Figure 5.4 Electrode configuration for measuring standard electrode potential.

TABLE 5.1 STANDARD ELECTROCHEMICAL POTENTIALS AT 25°C

Lithium	−3.02	$Li^+ + e^- = Li$
Potassium	−2.92	$K^+ + e^- = K$
Sodium	−2.71	$Na^+ + e^- = Na$
Aluminum	−1.67	$Al^{+++} + 3e^- = Al$
Zinc	−0.762	$Zn^{++} + 2e^- = Zn$
Iron	−0.440	$Fe^{++} + 2e^- = Fe$
Cadmium	−0.402	$Cd^{++} + 2e^- = Cd$
Hydrogen	0.000	$2H^+ + 2e^- = H_2$
Copper	0.337	$Cu^{++} + 2e^- = Cu$
Silver	0.7991	$Ag^+ + e^- = Ag$
Mercury	0.852	$Hg^{++} + 2e^- = Hg$
Oxygen	1.229	$O_2 + 4H^+ + 4e^- = 2H_2O$
Chlorine	1.356	$Cl_2 + 2e^- = 2Cl^-$

that when zinc metal is placed in a solution of HCl, hydrogen is produced. When copper metal is placed in a solution of HCl, the copper is polished. No hydrogen is produced.

Typical standard electrochemical potentials are shown in Table 5.1.

REFERENCE ELECTRODES

The standard hydrogen electrode (SHE) is difficult to maintain accurately, and several alternate electrodes are used as reference electrodes in potential measurements. These consist of a metal in equilibrium with a slightly soluble salt. The salts are usually chlorides, and a solution of potassium chloride covers the salt. The concentration of potassium chloride in the cell affects the potential. The *saturated calomel electrode* (SCE) contains a saturated solution of potassium chloride:

$$Hg_2Cl_2 + 2e^- = 2Hg + 2Cl^- \qquad E = 0.246 \text{ volts}$$

The *normal calomel electrode* contains a 1 N solution of potassium chloride and has the same equation as the previous one but $E = 0.280$ volts.

The *normal silver–silver chloride* electrode half-cell equation is

$$AgCl + e^- = Ag + Cl^- \qquad E = 0.237 \text{ volts}$$

THE NERNST EQUATION

When the concentrations in a cell differ from those required for the standard electrode potential, the Nernst equation (derivable from basic thermodynamic notions of free energy) provides a means of calculating the potential:

$$E = E_o - \frac{RT}{nF} \ln \frac{(\text{Red.})}{(\text{Ox.})}$$

For standard body conditions (37°C) the coefficient, using common logarithms (to the base 10) instead of ln to the base e, becomes 0.061

$$E = E_o - 0.061 \log (\text{Red.})/(\text{Ox.})$$

MEASUREMENT OF pH

Since pH $= -\log[H^+]$, and E_o for hydrogen $= 0.0$, the measurement of hydrogen ion potential will provide the pH directly from the electrode, $E_{pH} = -0.061 \log[H^+]$. The glass electrode is the common electrode for the measurement of pH. This electrode uses a glass membrane which is a "specific-ion electrode"; it reacts with the hydrogen ion and with (almost) no other ion. As the hydrogen ion approaches the outside of the electrode, the silicate structure of the glass acts like a solid-state P-conductor, conducting the positive charges (holes) into the internal solution, which contains a metal–metal oxide electrode (SCE or Ag/AgCl). A reference electrode must also be inserted into the solution to provide a measured potential against which the pH potential is compared by a pH meter (a VTVM designed for high input impedance). The impedance of the pH electrode can be of the magnitude of 10 to 100 megohms.

CONDUCTIMETRIC MEASUREMENTS

If potentiometry is primarily a voltage measurement, conductimetry is primarily a current measurement, but electrolytic conduction differs from electronic conduction. In conduction through a wire, electrons are moving in the electron cloud that constitutes the inside of most metallic structures. Conduction through a solution consists of the motion of ions, positive ions in one direction and negative ions in the other. When arriving at the electrodes, the ions may undergo some chemical change which may generate a potential and provide potentiometric interference with the current measurement.

Faraday's laws of electrochemical equivalence, which he published in 1883 and 1884, have come down through the years unchanged. His laws state that 1) the amount of chemical change produced by a current is directly proportional to the quantity of electricity passing through the solution; and 2) the amount of substance liberated by a current is directly proportional to the equivalent weight of the material.

Combined, the laws state that one electrochemical equivalent of a substance is formed by the passage of one *faraday* of electricity. One faraday is equal to 96,500 coulombs. Hence, there is a direct connection between current flow and material deposited. In fact, before the present system of standards was adopted, the standard for coulomb was the amount of electricity necessary to deposit 0.00111800 grams of silver, and this weight is of course the equivalent weight of silver divided by 96,500 coulombs per equivalent weight.

A coulometer is a device that uses the principle just described to measure the total current flow. The coulometer is placed in the electrical circuit, and at the end of the desired period the silver deposited is weighed, providing an accurate measure of the total current flow.

The flow through an electrolyte is a flow through a *volume*, and provides difficulty for those of us who think of flow through a wire as a linear flow. Thus, the first quantities to be standardized are the shape and extent of the volume. A cube consisting of two flat parallel electrodes, each 1 cm. square and located 1 cm. from each other, is the standard volume. The resistance of a material filling that standard volume is called the specific resistance of the material, the reciprocal of which is the standard conductance, $K = 1/R$. One gram-equivalent of an electrolyte dissolved in water in this standard volume is the standard amount of material the resistance of which is to be measured. The equivalent conductance is the conductance of 1 gram-equivalent weight of material dissolved in 1 liter of water.

The equation for resistance measured by an electrode is

$$R = r \left(\frac{L}{A}\right) \quad \text{in ohms}$$

where r = specific resistance

L = length of cell

A = cross-sectional area of cell

Rather than measuring L and A, a solution is used whose resistance is known, and L/A is considered to be the cell constant.

Equivalent Conductance $(\Omega) = 1000$ k/C in ohms per g.-eqt. per cm^3, C = concentration in g.-eqt. per 1000 cm^3, and k = specific conductance in ohms per cm.

CARRIERS OF CURRENT IN AN IONIC SOLUTION

When two electrodes are placed in an ionic solution and a potential is applied, if the potential is great enough, a current will flow. If a DC meter is attached to the circuit, the current will be observed to increase to a maximum and then decrease to zero. An accumulation of positive ions has collected around the negative electrode, and an accumulation of negative ions has accumulated around the positive electrode. The driving potential of the electrodes is no longer felt in the body of the solution, and the cell has been polarized. Hence, conductance in a solution is much different from conductance in a wire. The ions that conduct the current are themselves charged; in their motion through the solution they pass through a charged field, and when they arrive at the electrodes, they produce a charged field in the solution opposite in sign to that possessed by the electrodes.

Transference is the process whereby the current is carried by the

TABLE 5.2 EQUIVALENT IONIC CONDUCTANCE AT INFINITE DILUTION (25°C)

Potassium	73.52
Sodium	50.11
Ammonium	74.5
Silver	63.5
½Barium	65.0
½Calcium	60.0
Chloride	75.5
Nitrate	70.6
Acetate	40.8
½Sulfate	79.0
½Oxalate	73.0
Hydrogen ion	350.0
Hydroxyl ion	192.0

moving ions. The transference number of an ion is the fraction of the total current carried by that ion, or

$$t_- = \frac{I_-}{I}$$

where I = total current carried

t_- = transference number of negative ion

I_- = actual current carried by the negative ion

Thus, the equivalent conductance of the negative ion in this solution would be $\Omega_- = t_-\Omega$, the transference number times the total equivalent conductance of the salt (Table 5.2). The transference number of an ion can be measured independently of the conductance. Hence, the specific ionic conductance can be calculated for each ion and the total conductance of a salt calculated from the ionic conductances of its constituent ions.

From Table 5.2 the values shown in Table 5.3 may be derived.

The preceding discussion is absolutely accurate only at infinite dilution in which the Debye-Huckel and Onsager-Fuoss ionic cloud has no effect on ionic movement. The numbers are useful, however,

TABLE 5.3 CALCULATED EQUIVALENT CONDUCTANCE OF AQUEOUS SOLUTIONS VS. ACTUAL VALUES

Substance	Contributed by		Calculated Total	Actual Value
	Cation	Anion		
KCl	73.52	73.5	147.0	149.9
HCl	350.00	73.5	423.5	426.2
KNO$_3$	73.52	70.6	144.0	145.0
HNO$_3$	350.00	70.6	420.6	421.3
NaCl	50.11	73.5	123.6	126.5

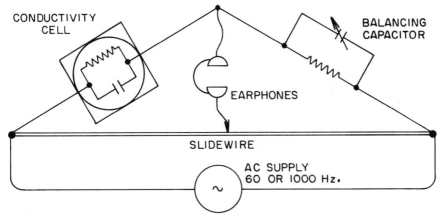

Figure 5.5 Modified Wheatstone bridge for conductance measurements of solutions.

for obtaining approximate results in real solutions, and in explaining the effect of various ions on the conductivity of solutions. Note how close the calculations are to the real values in Table 5.3.

METHODS OF MEASURING CURRENT IN SOLUTION

To avoid the polarization of the conductivity cell, AC bridges are used to measure the conductivity of solutions. As soon as a sinusoidal voltage is applied to a solution, the impedance of the solution electrode interface becomes important. Since conductivity is usually measured by a pair of parallel plates, the capacitance of this measuring device adds capacitive reactance to the resistance of the solution, obscuring the measurement. Hence, it is customary for analysts to add a capacitor in the balancing side of the bridge (Fig. 5.5).

The capacitor is adjusted until a minimum sound is heard in the earphones. (An AC meter or an "electric eye" is often used instead of the earphones; an oscilloscope would be the best detector.) The slide wire is moved until the earphone sound is reduced to a minimum. The balancing capacitor is readjusted, and the procedure repeated until the minimum signal is heard in the earphones. Figure 5.6 is

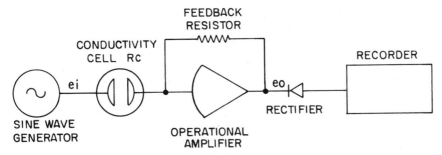

Figure 5.6 Operational amplifier conductivity measurement

an alternative approach to recording the conductivity of a cell, using an operational amplifier. The output of the operational amplifier is $e_o = -e_i(Z_f/Z_R)$. The diode in the output circuit will rectify the AC current to provide the DC current needed for the recorder. An adjustable capacitance in the feedback loop can be used to balance the capacitance of the cell with a reference solution in it.

The sine wave generator can be built with operational amplifiers by noting that if

$$y = A \sin Wt,$$

then

$$\frac{dy}{dt} = WA \cos Wt,$$

and

$$\frac{d^2y}{dt^2} = -W^2A \sin Wt = -W^2y.$$

This system can be implemented by the operational amplifier circuit.

POLAROGRAPHY

Polarography takes advantage of the polarization that occurs at the electrode when a current flows through a solution. By using a microelectrode, a diffusion-limited current can be produced, i.e., a current limited by the rate at which ions can diffuse from the body of the solution to the minute area of the electrode. By selecting the potential at which this diffusion-limited current is measured, one can determine the particular ions that will be moved in the solution. Thus, a qualitative analysis — dependent on the potential applied — and a quantitative analysis — dependent on the current obtained at that potential — can be provided.

Heyrovsky developed the polarograph, which provided just such an adjustable potential and derived the diffusion theory, which related the current obtained to the concentration of ions in solution. With such an instrument and modern technology, one can use a standard solution for calibration, thus eliminating all the errors which may occur in the application of the theory to a real solution.

STANDARD POLAROGRAPHIC INSTRUMENT

Heyrovsky used a dropping mercury electrode (DME) for his microelectrode. The mercury drop, while still hanging, provided a microsurface for his electrode; after it dropped, it provided a renewable surface which carried its polarized environment away with it. The term polarography has been associated with the DME, which cannot be used in biomedical studies. The term voltammetry is used for the general subject. The terms shall be used interchangeably for the purposes of this discussion. However, it should be kept in mind that we differ from the traditional electrochemist who uses polarography only for analyses with the DME.

The usual potential-meter is in the form of a slide wire connected across a calibrated potential source with a range of 0 to −1.2 volts, the DME being a cathode with respect to the standard calomel electrode. A vacuum-tube voltmeter is used to read the potential across the cell, without loading down the cell; an ammeter in series with the cell provides the current flow reading, which is in the order of microamperes. A typical voltage current curve is shown in Figure 5.7.

The midpoint of each polarographic wave is called the half-wave potential ($E_{1/2}$) and is characteristic of the E_0 standard electrode potential for that ion. Thus, in Figure 5.7 the half-wave potential for Pb is 0.5 volts, and that for Zn is 1.13 volts. The diffusion current is the difference between the current before the wave and after the wave. For Pb it would be $5.0 - 1.0 = 4.0$ microamperes. For Zn it would be $9.6 - 5.0 = 4.6$ microamperes. The height of each of these steps is related to concentration by a calibration curve such as that shown in Figure 5.8.

In addition to the sample to be analyzed, the polarographic cell must contain a supporting electrolyte, i.e., an electrolyte which will conduct the current but which will not be oxidized or reduced in the

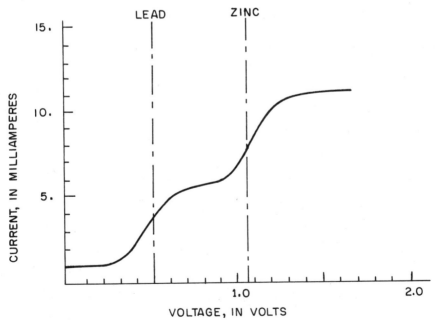

Figure 5.7 Typical polarographic current voltage curve.

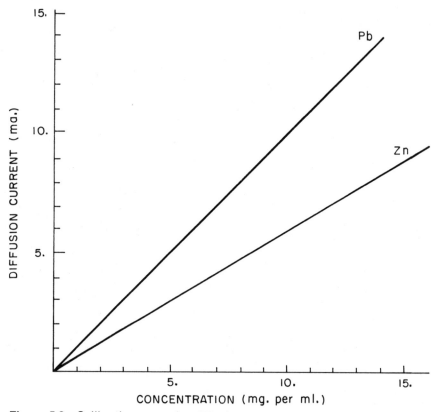

Figure 5.8 Calibration curve for diffusion current.

region of analysis. Typical supporting electrolytes are 1 M solutions of KCl, NH_3 in NH_4Cl, NaOH, and KCN. Also used is 7.3 M H_3PO_4. Dissolved oxygen interferes with polarograms at −0.05 volts (where oxygen is reduced to peroxide) and at −0.9 volts (where oxygen is reduced to water). In polarographic analyses, the oxygen is removed by bubbling nitrogen through the solution. In biomedical studies, it is oxygen that has to be determined.

BIOMEDICAL POLAROGRAPHIC APPLICATIONS

Clinical laboratory polarographic procedures using the DME detect the presence of sodium, potassium, lithium, lead, and other heavy metals in blood and other fluids directly. For live measurements of body fluids, however, a different procedure must be used. Instead of the DME, a platinum electrode is used. A flowing stream provides a self-renewable fluid, and hence compensates for one of the requirements of the microelectrode. The other requirement, its small dimension, can be met by providing a needle-point electrode. Because of the need for the applied potential, damage to body tissues might result. Hence, analyses of trace amounts of metallic materials and of anions such as phosphate and sulfate are provided for by the use of ion-selective potentiometric electrodes, to be described next. The principal application of polarography in biomedical instrumentation is the Clark electrode for oxygen.

DISSOLVED OXYGEN ELECTRODES

Two types of electrodes available for analysis of oxygen in body fluids are the Hersch cell and the Clark cell. The Hersch cell uses silver and lead electrodes in 24% potassium hydroxide electrolyte. The entire cell is contained in a polyethylene membrane, permeable to oxygen but not to larger molecules like proteins. As the oxygen diffuses into the cell, it permits a flow of current as the following electrode reactions take place. At the silver electrode, $O_2 + 2H_2O + 4e^- \rightleftharpoons 4OH^-$; the oxygen is reduced to hydroxide. At the lead electrode, $Pb + 2OH^- \rightleftharpoons Pb(OH)_2 + 2e^-$. The hydroxyl ion produced at the cathode diffuses through the cell to the lead anode where it produces lead hydroxide, soluble in the potassium hydroxide electrolyte. A current flow of 10 microamperes per part per million of oxygen is produced.

The Clark cell contains a platinum-measuring electrode and a reference electrode of silver/silver oxide in a potassium hydroxide electrolyte. Originally the membrane used was Teflon, but now polyethylene is being used. The oxygen-polarizing potential is applied across the cell, and the current flow is measured. The "diffusion current" measured is proportional to oxygen concentration in the surrounding fluid (or gas) in the p.p.m. range.

ION-SELECTIVE ELECTRODES

Having outlined the difficulties inherent in the analysis of biomedical substrates with potentiometric, conductimetric, and polarographic methods, we now approach the most modern member of the electrode series, the ion-selective electrode (Fig. 5.9). Like the glass electrode and the Clark electrode, the ion-selective electrode contains a membrane through which the specific ion diffuses more rapidly than any other ion, and an internal detection potentiometric system which is more sensitive to the particular ion that we desire to detect than to any other. The ion-selective electrode, although selective in its response, will respond to other ions.

The selectivity ratio is a measure of its preference for the ion of interest. The membrane can be regarded as an ion exchanger; it actively seeks the ion of interest and rejects to a variable extent all others. Thus, the glass electrode is selective to hydrogen ions but will also respond to sodium and potassium. By changes in glass composition it

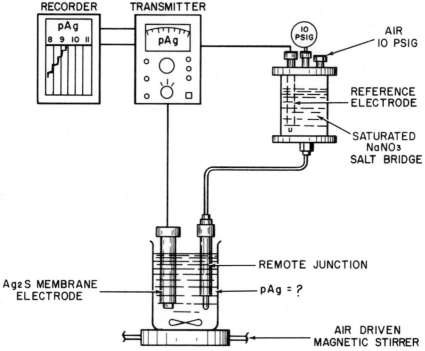

Figure 5.9 Typical ion selective measuring system. (From B. G. Lipták (ed.) *Instrument Engineers' Handbook* (Vol. II). Philadelphia: Chilton, 1970.)

can be made selective to sodium, potassium, thallium, lithium, or cesium. Liquid ion exchangers have been developed for anions such as iodide, bromide, chloride, and fluoride. A study of the cell membrane has made it possible to duplicate the selectivity of neutral membranes. In the preceding section we discussed the use of polyethylene and Teflon for oxygen analysis.

The use of silicone rubber as a binder material has provided heterogeneous membrane materials that hold ion-exchange resins, precipitates, carbides, borides, and silicides, and are sensitive to chloride, iodide, or sulfide. Reference electrodes are needed, as in normal potentiometric measurements. We have seen in our study of physiology that the calcium ion is important in biological fluids. An ion-exchange electrode with high specificity to calcium will be a very useful tool to biomedical instrumentalists. Finally, we shall discuss biomedical applications of glass electrodes for hydrogen ion and other cations, and of the other electrode types primarily for calcium.

SOLID ION EXCHANGERS

The glass electrode is an example of a solid ion exchanger. It is made from mixtures of oxides of silicon and aluminum with oxides of sodium and calcium. When melted and cooled, an amorphous crystalline material forms, crystalline in the trivalent cations and amorphous in the univalent cation. Hence, the monovalent charged ions are free to move in the trivalent crystalline membrane. If the membrane separates two fluids containing univalent ions, a Nernst potential is developed,

$$E = \frac{RT}{F} \ln \frac{a_i}{a_o}$$

where the a's represent the activities of the same univalent cation on the two sides of the membrane. The glass electrode is filled on the inside with a salt of constant composition (KCl), and the potential developed is thus a function of the univalent ion concentrations on the outside.

$$E = -(\text{const}) \log a_o$$

Hence, if the univalent ion on the outside is H^+ the potential measured is a function of the pH: $E = (\text{const}) \times pH$.

If Na^+ and K^+ are also present in the solution, the glass electrode will respond to them. By evolution, the composition of the glass electrode has been modified until the sensitivity to H^+ is much greater than to Na^+ or to K^+, and our present ion-selective pH glass electrode is the result of this development. By modifying the glass composition, glass electrodes have been built which are more sensitive to Na^+, and the potential measured is proportional to $-\log[Na^+]$, which is termed pNa. Glass formulations have also been made which are more selective for K^+ than for Na^+. The selectivity ratio is $10:1$, but this is sufficient for the determination of K^+ in kidney nephron tubular fluid, with the Na^+ electrode used as a reference.

MEMBRANE ELECTRODES

Membrane electrodes may consist of an inactive membrane holding an active liquid or a solid state ion exchange material. Liquid ion exchangers contain a liquid ion exchange material held in a Millipore filter with pore diameter of about 100 millimicrons. Esters of phosphoric acid have high selectivity for calcium ion (Ross, in Durst [1969]). Other liquid membrane systems have been developed for copper, lead, nitrate, chloride, and chlorate.

Solid-State Membranes

A lanthanum fluoride membrane electrode has been developed for detection of fluoride ion. Silver sulfide is used as a sulfide ion detector. Silver halides dispersed in silver sulfide provide a chloride–bromide electrode: silver chloride in silver sulfide is an electrode sensitive to chloride ion; silver bromide in silver sulfide electrode is sensitive to bromide ion; and silver iodide in silver sulfide is sensitive to iodide ion.

The use of metallic sulfides in the silver sulfide matrix provides cation-sensitive electrodes. Copper sulfide produces a copper-sensitive electrode; lead sulfide produces a lead-sensitive electrode; and cadmium sulfide produces a cadmium-sensitive electrode. The solid-state membrane is very specific, since it provides an electrode response only if it is in contact with the material to which it is sensitive, except that anything that reacts with the solid will interfere with its response. Thus, thiocyanate ion will react with silver bromide and reduce its electrode potential.

The solid-state membranes are more selective than the organic liquid membranes. Conversely, the liquid organic membranes are more versatile, and can be developed for almost any cation or anion. When it is not possible to find a solid material in the proper crystalline form to make a solid-state membrane electrode, it may be possible to disperse the required material in an inert binder to form a heterogeneous membrane electrode that *will* do the job.

HETEROGENEOUS MEMBRANE ELECTRODES

Silicone rubber is the most popular binder for the ion-exchange material in the heterogeneous membrane electrode. Polystyrene, polyethylene, and polyvinyl chloride have also been used. In this inactive binder, active materials such as ion-exchange resins and precipitates have been dispersed. The most popular ion-exchange resin was Amberlite IR 120, which when dispersed in polystyrene and wetted with sodium chloride solution provided a sodium ion response. Pungor prepared ion-exchange resins sensitive to sulfate, chloride, hydroxide, hydrogen, potassium, zinc, and nickel. Precipitates such as calcium oxalate, barium sulfate, the silver halides, and calcium and lanthanum fluorides have been tried.

Silver halides have been successfully used and are available commercially (Hungary) for iodide, bromide, chloride, and sulfide. Barium sulfate and bismuth phosphate have been used for detection of sulfate and phosphate ions. Chloride ions above 10^{-3} M interfere with phosphate ions. The phosphate electrode appeared originally to have extensive drift, but this was a test of an early prototype. Sulfide electrodes have been constructed of silver sulfide in silicone rubber.

BIOMEDICAL APPLICATIONS OF ION-SELECTIVE ELECTRODES

Ion-selective electrodes for sodium, potassium, and calcium have provided extensive advancement in the study of biomedical systems. Biological systems are affected by ionic activities rather than by ionic concentrations. Potentiometric measurements, however, measure exactly the ionic activity that is of interest to biomedical researchers and medical practitioners. Electrodes can be inserted into living tissues to measure the active ion potentials, rather than resort being made to the clinical technique of removing a fluid sample and expecting the later clinical analysis to represent the actual condition in the system. Dynamic changes in the system can be noted as a matter of course with in situ electrodes, whereas in taking individual samples, the same detection would require a stroke of luck.

The Na^+-sensitive and K^+-sensitive glass electrodes are available in microelectrode form which can be inserted directly into tissues for measuring sodium and potassium concentrations. The pH microelectrode can measure the pH of blood in a 25 microliter sample to an accuracy of ± 0.006 pH units (Khuri, in Durst, 1969). Clinical analysis of urine and gastric samples are also common.

In situ measurements have been made of the pH and cation activity in the single proximal tubule of the nephron of the kidney. Glass pH microelectrodes were used to measure the pH, and the Na^+ microelectrode to measure $[Na^+]$, i.e., pNa. A reference micropipet filled with 3 M RbCl was used because of the extremely small response of the Na^+ microelectrode to Rb^+. Measurements of intercellular ionic activities of H^+, Na^+, K^+, and Cl^- have been measured in the protoplasm of single fibers of nerve and muscle, and the alga *Nitella*.

Fluoride ion has been measured in serum, mineralized tissue, saliva, toothpastes, and mouthwashes. Evidence was obtained for two forms of fluoride in human serum.

BIOMEDICAL STUDIES WITH CALCIUM ELECTRODES

Moore (in Durst, 1969) presents an extensive survey of biomedical studies which have been recently performed with ion-selective electrodes. He points out that 35 years ago it was proved that ionized calcium is the physiologically active species. Bone formation, nerve conduction, muscle contraction, cardiac activity, cerebral function, renal function, intestinal secretion, blood coagulation, membrane permeability, enzyme function, and hormonal release may all be dependent on calcium ion concentration. The availability of the calcium ion-exchange electrode has made this area of research accessible to the scientist.

Moore performed an analysis of calcium in serum, which is in equilibrium with the calcium of bone, cartilage, kidney, and intestine. There are three forms of calcium in serum including 1.) protein-bound type, which is nondiffusible; 2.) diffusible but nonionized complexed or chelated Ca^{++} (CaR); and 3.) ionized calcium. In normal man the third type is maintained at close tolerances. The pH of venous blood is 7.34 ± 0.01, whereas the pH of separated serum is 7.42 ± 0.01. Moore found that the serum total calcium levels normally measured in hospitals correlate closely with serum albumin, while the ionized calcium measured with the electrodes is relatively constant in normal subjects. In normal subjects, serum calcium levels are between 2.25 and 2.75 millimoles (mM.); serum ionized calcium levels are 1.16 mM.; CaR levels are 0.3 mM. In patients with malignancy and hypercalcemia, increase in total serum calcium was accompanied by a rise in ionized calcium to maintain 45% of total, and by a rise of protein-bound calcium to maintain 44%. The model was developed for the state of serum calcium in normal subjects and cirrhotic patients, as well as in patients with hypercalcemia owing to malignancy.

The ion-exchange electrodes, although still not small enough to insert into the body, proved very useful in studying the calcium concentration of serum removed from the patients under study.

SUMMARY

Electrochemistry is an essential tool in the study of living systems. The study of ions in solution involves electrical phenomena produced by the ions, such as potential and current flow, which can be readily measured by current electrical techniques if the special properties of solutions are borne in mind. The equilibrium constants of ions in solution based on Guldberg and Waage's mass action law provide K_{SP} for slightly soluble salts, K_i for slightly ionized acids and bases, and K_w as the ion product of water, the basis of all acid and base measurements. All the principles of electrochemistry hold accurately at infinite dilution, the activity coefficient providing a means for using the principles in real solutions. The measurement of the oxidation-reduction potential of ions in solution is termed potentiometry. It can be performed by electrodes which are reversible and is measured by relative potential related to the potential of the standard hydrogen electrode.

Other standard reference electrodes are used because of the difficulty of making a reproducible hydrogen gas electrode. The saturated and normal calomel electrodes are used as such references. The Nernst equation is a mathematical representation of the potential obtained from an oxidation-reduction electrode. The measurement of pH can be said to be performed by such an electrode, although the glass electrode appears to be an inert nonreactive device.

Conductimetric measurements involve the measurement of the flow of current in a solution. The current is carried by the ions, not all ions carrying the same amount, and the transference number is a measure of the ratio of the total current carried by each ion. In order to avoid the ions accumulating around the electrodes and polarizing the solution, an alternating voltage is used to measure the current flow in solution. Polarography uses the polarization that occurs at the electrode with direct current flow to measure the concentration of that ion in solution. Both qualitative and quantitative measurements can be made by polarography. The half-wave potential is characteristic of the individual ion, and the wave height is characteristic of the concentration of that individual ion. Biomedical application of polarography is confined to the measurement of dissolved oxygen, although many organic materials can be analyzed by this method.

Ion-selective electrodes comprise the new interesting topic in electrochemistry that is exciting the biomedical specialist. A selective membrane is coupled with a selective electrode to provide the selectivity required to make potentiometric measurements of vital fluids. The membrane is inert except for the solid-state membrane, which is a pure crystal of a salt that will allow only the ions in that salt through the membrane.

The glass electrode is a type of solid-state electrode, but it is not specific—it can be made selective for hydrogen, sodium, or potassium ions. A finely pored filter holding an organic phosphate is used as an ion-selective membrane for calcium. A heterogeneous membrane consists of a silicone rubber binder and a precipitate, or ion-exchange resin. Ion-selective electrodes have been used in biomedical studies and are beginning to be used in the study of in situ electrode placement for determination of sodium, potassium, and pH, and in the external study of blood serum and the calcium in the tissues.

EXERCISES

1. The solubility product of silver chloride is 1.8×10^{-10}. What would be the concentration of silver ion and of chloride ion in a solution prepared by shaking a 0.01 M solution of $AgNO_3$ with a 0.01 M solution of HCl?

2. The dissociation constant of HAc is 1.75×10^{-5}. What will be the pH of a solution of 10^{-4} N HAc? If the solution is made 0.01 N with respect to NaAc, what would be the pH?

3. Using Table 5.2, what would be the potential of each of the following electrode configurations:

     a. $Al/Al^{+++}//Ag^+/Ag$;   b. $Zn/Zn^{++}//Cu^{++}/Cu$;

     c. $Cd/Cd^{++}//Zn^{++}/Zn$;   d. $Al/Al^{+++}//Cd^{++}/Cd$

4. What would be the Nernst potential generated by a cell containing 0.01 N Fe^{++} and 0.001 N Fe^{+++}?

5. Using Table 5.2, what would be the specific conductance of 3 N KCl? What reading in mhos would be obtained in a cell with a cell constant of 0.5?

6. Using Figure 5.8 as the correct calibration curve for a polarographic analysis of Pb and Zn in blood serum, what would be the concentration of these two metals in 100 ml. of serum, if the diffusion current for the Pb peak was 5 ma., and that for the Zn peak was 7.5 ma.?

7. A Clark cell is inserted in a blood vessel, and a current of 2.5 ma. is

measured. Calibration of the cell produces a curve identical with that shown in Figure 5.8 for Pb. Calculate the oxygen concentration in mg. per ml. of blood.

8. A sodium-sensitive glass electrode is placed into a blood vessel and connected to a pH meter which reads a millivoltage corresponding to a pH of 7 against a silver–silver chloride reference electrode. What is the concentration of Na^{++} in the subject's blood if the same reference electrode is used?

9. A pH microelectrode is inserted into a nephron of a living kidney, and a reading of 4.5 is observed. Use the information in this chapter to compute the bicarbonate concentration in the measured vessel.

10. Devise a system for the mass screening of incipient cancer in man using the data given in the section describing the calcium electrode.

General Literature Cited and References

Durst, R. A. (editor) Ion Selective Electrodes. *NBS Special Publication, 314:* 1969.

Geddes, L. A., and Baker, L. E. Principles of Applied Biomedical Instrumentation. New York: Wiley, 1968.

MacInnes, D. A. The Principles of Electrochemistry. New York: Dover, 1961.

Meites, L., and Thomas, H. C. Advanced Analytical Chemistry. New York: McGraw-Hill, 1958.

Operational amplifiers symposium. *Anal. Chem. 35:* 1770, 1963.

Plonsey, R., and Fleming, D. Bioelectric Phenomena. New York: McGraw-Hill, 1969.

Weiss, M. D. Electrochemical Methods in Process Controls. Proceedings of the 6th Instrumental Analysis Symposium, ISA, 1960.

Chapter 6

Physical Methods of Analysis

IN ADDITION TO electrochemistry, many other methods of analysis are available for biomedical studies. The electromagnetic spectrum provides 22 decades of electromagnetic energy which can be absorbed preferentially by desired species of molecules to provide useful analysis of biological fluids. Chromatography is an analytical method for separating gases or liquids, which can be used with instrumental detection techniques to provide a better understanding of biological materials. X-ray and electron microscopy have become the tools of the molecular biologist, helping him to understand the biological building blocks. All these techniques are evolving from the research laboratory to the hospital, clinic, and physician's office and provide improved methods of detecting disease and abnormalities in human tissue and fluids.

THE FREQUENCY SPECTRUM

Before measuring instruments were available to assist the physician in diagnosing the patient's condition, he relied solely on his senses to furnish clues of systemic abnormalities. Smell, taste, feel, sound, and sight were utilized. The smell of acetone on the patient's breath, e.g., is a symptom of diabetes mellitus. A sweet taste in urine (glycosuria), the color (pallor?) of the skin, tenseness in the abdomen, and irregular heart sounds all make direct use of the physician's senses.

A glance at Figure 6.1 shows that the sense of sight, e.g., can be extended by a factor of 10^{22} by use of the electromagnetic spectrum.

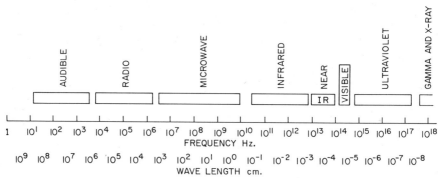

Figure 6.1 The frequency spectrum.

Looking at the frequency spectrum, we see DC and AC in the 0 to 100 Hz. region, the first two decades. Electrochemical analysis including the galvanic cell measuring redox potential and pH, and the conductivity analyzers operating at 60 Hz., can be placed in this region.

From 60 to 1000 Hz. we have the impedance measurements, electrical measurements that are dependent on frequency. The audible region of the spectrum from 10 Hz. to 10,000 Hz. includes the range of high fidelity equipment, the physician's stethoscope, and sonic and ultrasonic analyzers. These will be discussed in Chapters 8 and 9.

From 10^4 to 10^7 includes the region of radiowaves (10 to 1000 kHz.), and the microwave region 1 mega-Hz. and beyond. Here, the spin of the atom and the nucleus give analytical information, and we can demonstrate nuclear magnetic resonance and electron paramagnetic resonance. Finally, we arrived at 10^{11} to 10^{14} Hz.—the infrared region. Here are electromagnetic waves like our visible rays, but unfortunately they are not detectable without special instrumentation. From 10^{14} to 10^{15} is the one decade available to man's range of vision. Here we have developed colorimeters, spectrometers, interferometers, and holographic instruments, image intensifiers, and the television tube—even the color television tube—to assist our limited vision and extend our horizons a few tenths of a decade in the visible region. Then in the decades, 10^{15} to 10^{17} (ultraviolet region), molecular spectra appear, and double bonds provide information. The X-ray region (10^{16} to 10^{19}) provides information about the crystalline structure of matter and the variation in density of organic materials. The gamma region (10^{17} to 10^{22}) is where nuclear measurements can be made, using radioactive tracers. Beyond 10^{22} lies the range of cosmic radiation, now detectable by the astronauts as they travel through space.

Each of these regions has been investigated by schools of physicists at different times in history. In each region, sources and detectors

TABLE 6.1 PHYSICAL DEVICES FOR INSTRUMENTATION OF THE FREQUENCY SPECTRUM

Range	Source	Detector
sonic	vibratory	microphone
radio frequency	radio frequency generator	tuned circuit
microwave	klystron	resonant cavity
infrared	hot body	bolometer
visible	lamp	photocell
ultraviolet	ultraviolet lamp	ultraviolet phototube
X-ray	X-ray tube	Geiger-Müller counter
gamma	radioactive	scintillation counter; scaler

have been developed, and special materials have been found or invented to conduct the energy required. Table 6.1 outlines some of the sources and detectors developed in each region. These instruments were used in the physical and chemical research laboratory, but because of their delicacy were not very useful for routine clinical laboratory purposes or for bedside monitoring.

Next, the gas chromatograph was developed in the 1950's for use in routine clinical laboratories. It consists of a separating column followed either by one of the physical methods of detection listed in Table 6.1 or the measurement of the thermal conductivity of the gas in the detector. The column provides a qualitative separation, and the detector a quantitative analysis of each qualitative fraction.

Lastly, the "chemist in the box" was developed, utilizing automated analysis. Automated processes were used for example to separate the components in a blood sample, and physical methods were used to obtain a rapid, easily transduced quantitative signal for each component.

SPECTROMETRIC METHODS OF ANALYSIS

Spectrometric methods of analysis include all methods of analysis of matter based on interactions of the matter with electromagnetic energy. We shall end our study in this section of the text at the radio-frequency end of the spectrum, at about 10^5 Hz. Conductivity at the lowest end of the spectrum was discussed in Chapter 4. A study of the audible and ultrasonic regions of the spectrum involves special considerations and will be taken up in Chapter 7. The spectrometric portion of the spectrum usually includes the "colored" portion, i.e., radio, micro, infrared, visible, and ultraviolet waves. Radiation shorter in wavelength and higher in frequency than ultraviolet, such as X-rays, will be covered; nuclear emissions such as gamma rays, particles such as alpha and beta rays will be covered under nuclear instrumentation; the separation of charged ions by electric magnetic fields will be discussed in mass spectrometry; and the separation by physicochemical affinity will be taken up under chromatography.

Interaction of matter with electromagnetic energy can assume several forms. The energy can be absorbed or diffracted, or cause fluorescence of the sample. The sample can be activated to emit a spectrum, which can be studied by a spectrometer, or recorded (usually photographically) by a spectrograph; or a spectrophotometer can measure the intensity of energy transmitted or absorbed at specific dispersed wavelengths. A photometer may measure the total energy transmitted or absorbed in a given spectral region without dispersing the energy over individual wavelengths (nondispersive analysis).

Before we discuss these details, however, we need to understand the nature of electromagnetic energy and its interaction with matter.

ELECTROMAGNETIC ENERGY

James Clark Maxwell in 1873 proposed the hypothesis that light is propagated by an oscillating electrical field, which by its oscillations produces an induced magnetic field perpendicular to it. These properties explained the concepts of reflection, refraction, diffraction, interference, and polarization present in all forms of "electromagnetic" energy from radiowaves to cosmic radiation. Quantum mechanics shows that radiant energy has a dual nature—it has properties of waves, but it can also be quantized as photons or packets of energy. In spectrometric methods of analysis we use the wave nature of light to control it in the instrument and the photon nature of light to explain its interaction with matter.

Light, or radiant energy, if we want to extend our discussion beyond the visible spectrum, has properties like frequency (v), wavelength (λ), and velocity (c), which are related as follows:

$$c = v\lambda$$

The wavelength is the distance between adjacent peaks of the oscillatory wave, and the frequency is the number of oscillations per second of the wave; hence, the product of the two is the velocity with which the wave is propagated. The energy content of radiation is derived from the packet principle and was found by Planck (and Einstein) to be proportional to the frequency

$$E = hv$$

where h = Planck's constant = 6.62×10^{-27} erg seconds, and
  c = velocity of light = 3.00×10^{10} cm. per second in vacuo.

The regions of electromagnetic energy shown in Figure 6.1 are

TABLE 6.2 UNITS OF ELECTROMAGNETIC SPECTRUM

One	Meter	Centimeter	Millimeter	Micron	Millimicron
Angstrom	10^{-10}	10^{-8}	10^{-7}	10^{-4}	0.1
Millimicron	10^{-9}	10^{-7}	10^{-6}	10^{-3}	1.0
Micron	10^{-6}	10^{-4}	10^{-3}	1.0	1000
Millimeter	10^{-3}	10^{-1}	1.0	1000	10^6
Meter	1.0	100	1000	10^6	10^9

characterized by their wavelength, and different units have developed in each region of energy. Thus, X-rays are expressed in Angstrom units (Å), ultraviolet and visible radiation in millimicrons (mμ), infrared radiation in microns (μ), microwaves in centimeters (cm.), and radiowaves in meters (m.), although radiowaves are also characterized by their frequency in Hertz (Hz.) which are cycles per second. Table 6.2 outlines the relationship between the units.

THE NATURE OF MATTER

Radiant energy emitted in packets as derived from the equation $E = h\nu$ is also absorbed in similar quantized packets. The wavelength and frequency of the energy absorbed are functions of the structure of the matter. Hence, spectral analysis is the use of appropriate instrumentation to detect the critical wavelengths of radiant energy with which the particular structure of the sample is interacting. The nature of this interaction may be in the atoms of the molecule, an inner electron shift in the X-ray region, an outer electron shift in the ultraviolet or visible region, or a property of the molecule as a whole. The molecule may absorb a quantum of energy that would make it vibrate (near infrared), or rotate (far infrared). The energy of motion of the molecule as a whole is represented in the temperature of the material.

The Bohr-Rutherford concept of the atom although superseded by the modern quantum theory, gives a clear picture of the origin of spectra. In this atom there is a nucleus surrounded by a series of electrons in circular orbits. In modern terminology, the orbits of the planetary atom are called energy levels, and circular orbits are now called elliptical orbits characterized by an azimuthal quantum number k, as well as by the principal quantum number n. Two other quantum numbers complete the description of individual electrons: l, related to the rotation of the elliptical orbit about the nucleus; and m, related to the magnetic spin of the electron. With these four quantum numbers, one can proceed through the periodic table from hydrogen (at. no. 1) to lawrencium (at. no. 103) and assign s, p, d, f, and g quantum levels to each electron. (The mnemonic device students pray daily for (high) grades is used to remember the symbols for the quantum levels.)

PERIODIC TABLE

Thus, the Bohr-Rutherford atom has been replaced by the quantum energy level diagram (Fig. 6.2). The Bohr-Rutherford atom did not provide all the different energy levels required to represent the spectra obtained when electrons jump from one orbit to another. The

Atomic No.	Element	K 1 s	L 2 s p	M 3 s p d	N 4 s p d f	O 5 s p d f	P 6 s p d f	Q 7 s p d f
1	H	1						
2	He	2						
3	Li	2	1					
4	Be	2	2					
5	B	2	2 1					
6	C	2	2 2					
7	N	2	2 3					
8	O	2	2 4					
9	F	2	2 5					
10	Ne	2	2 6					
11	Na	2	2 6	1				
12	Mg	2	2 6	2				
13	Al	2	2 6	2 1				
14	Si	2	2 6	2 2				
15	P	2	2 6	2 3				
16	S	2	2 6	2 4				
17	Cl	2	2 6	2 5				
18	Ar	2	2 6	2 6				
19	K	2	2 6	2 6 ..	1			
20	Ca	2	2 6	2 6 ..	2			
21	Sc	2	2 6	2 6 1	2			
22	Ti	2	2 6	2 6 2	2			
23	V	2	2 6	2 6 3	2			
24	Cr	2	2 6	2 6 5*	1			
25	Mn	2	2 6	2 6 5	2			
26	Fe	2	2 6	2 6 6	2			
27	Co	2	2 6	2 6 7	2			
28	Ni	2	2 6	2 6 8	2			
29	Cu	2	2 6	2 6 10*	1			
30	Zn	2	2 6	2 6 10	2			
31	Ga	2	2 6	2 6 10	2 1			
32	Ge	2	2 6	2 6 10	2 2			
33	As	2	2 6	2 6 10	2 3			
34	Se	2	2 6	2 6 10	2 4			
35	Br	2	2 6	2 6 10	2 5			
36	Kr	2	2 6	2 6 10	2 6			
37	Rb	2	2 6	2 6 10	2 6 ..	1		
38	Sr	2	2 6	2 6 10	2 6 ..	2		
39	Y	2	2 6	2 6 10	2 6 1	2		
40	Zr	2	2 6	2 6 10	2 6 2 ..	2		
41	Nb	2	2 6	2 6 10	2 6 4*..	1		
42	Mo	2	2 6	2 6 10	2 6 5 ..	1		
43	Tc	2	2 6	2 6 10	2 6 6 ..	1		
44	Ru	2	2 6	2 6 10	2 6 7 ..	1		
45	Rh	2	2 6	2 6 10	2 6 8 ..	1		
46	Pd	2	2 6	2 6 10	2 6 10*..	0		
47	Ag	2	2 6	2 6 10	2 6 10 ..	1		
48	Cd	2	2 6	2 6 10	2 6 10 ..	2		
49	In	2	2 6	2 6 10	2 6 10 ..	2 1		
50	Sn	2	2 6	2 6 10	2 6 10 ..	2 2		
51	Sb	2	2 6	2 6 10	2 6 10 ..	2 3		
52	Te	2	2 6	2 6 10	2 6 10 ..	2 4		
53	I	2	2 6	2 6 10	2 6 10 ..	2 5		
54	Xe	2	2 6	2 6 10	2 6 10 ..	2 6		

* Note irregularity.

Figure 6.2 Electronic configuration of the elements. (From R. C. Weast (ed.) *Handbook of Chemistry and Physics* (51st ed.). Cleveland: The Chemical Rubber Co., 1970–1971.)

By Laurence S. Foster. References: F. H. Spedding and A. H. Duane, editors, *The Rare Earths,* John Wiley and

quantum mechanics atom with its multilevel energies on each principal energy level does provide enough levels so that any spectral line can be found from the equation $E_1 - E_2 = h\nu$.

When the procedure of placing the proper electrons in the proper shells is followed, not only do the predicted spectral data match the

Atomic No	Element	K 1 s	L 2 s p	M 3 s p d	N 4 s p d f	O 5 s p d f	P 6 s p d f	Q 7 s p d f
55	Cs	2	2 6	2 6 10	2 6 10 ..	2 6	1	
56	Ba	2	2 6	2 6 10	2 6 10 ..	2 6	2	
57	La	2	2 6	2 6 10	2 6 10 .	2 6 1 ..	2	
58	Ce	2	2 6	2 6 10	2 6 10 2*	2 6	2	
59	Pr	2	2 6	2 6 10	2 6 10 3	2 6	2	
60	Nd	2	2 6	2 6 10	2 6 10· 4	2 6	2	
61	Pm	2	2 6	2 6 10	2 6 10 5	2 6	2	
62	Sm	2	2 6	2 6 10	2 6 10 6	2 6	2	
63	Eu	2	2 6	2 6 10	2 6 10 7	2 6	2	
64	Gd	2	2 6	2 6 10	2 6 10 7	2 6 1 ..	2	
65	Tb	2	2 6	2 6 10	2 6 10 9*	2 6	2	
66	Dy	2	2 6	2 6 10	2 6 10 10	2 6	2	
67	Ho	2	2 6	2 6 10	2 6 10 11	2 6	2	
68	Er	2	2 6	2 6 10	2 6 10 12	2 6	2	
69	Tm	2	2 6	2 6 10	2 6 10 13	2 6	2	
70	Yb	2	2 6	2 6 10	2 6 10 14	2 6	2	
71	Lu	2	2 6	2 6 10	2 6 10 14	2 6 1 ..	2	
72	Hf	2	2 6	2 6 10	2 6 10 14	2 6 2 ..	2	
73	Ta	2	2 6	2 6 10	2 6 10 14	2 6 3 ..	2	
74	W	2	2 6	2 6 10	2 6 10 14	2 6 4 ..	2	
75	Re	2	2 6	2 6 10	2 6 10 14	2 6 5 ..	2	
76	Os	2	2 6	2 6 10	2 6 10 14	2 6 6 ..	2	
77	Ir	2	2 6	2 6 10	2 6 10 14	2 6 9* ..	0	
78	Pt	2	2 6	2 6 10	2 6 10 14	2 6 9 ..	1	
79	Au	2	2 6	2 6 10	2 6 10 14	2 6 10 ..	1	
80	Hg	2	2 6	2 6 10	2 6 10 14	2 6 10 ..	2	
81	Ti	2	2 6	2 6 10	2 6 10 14	2 6 10 ..	2 1	
82	Pb	2	2 6	2 6 10	2 6 10 14	2 6 10 ..	2 2	
83	Bi	2	2 6	2 6 10	2 6 10 14	2 6 10 ..	2 3	
84	Po	2	2 6	2 6 10	2 6 10 14	2 6 10 ..	2 4	
85	At	2	2 6	2 6 10	2 6 10 14	2 6 10 ..	2 5	
86	Rn	2	2 6	2 6 10	2 6 10 14	2 6 10 ..	2 6	
87	Fr	2	2 6	2 6 10	2 6 10 14	2 6 10 ..	2 6.. ..	1
88	Ra	2	2 6	2 6 10	2 6 10 14	2 6 10 ..	2 6.. ..	2
89	Ac	2	2 6	2 6 10	2 6 10 14	2 6 10 ..	2 6 1 ..	2
90	Th	2	2 6	2 6 10	2 6 10 14	2 6 10 ..	2 6 2 ..	2
91	Pa	2	2 6	2 6 10	2 6 10 14	2 6 10 2*	2 6 1 ..	2
92	U	2	2 6	2 6 10	2 6 10 14	2 6 10 3	2 6 1 ..	2
93	Np	2	2 6	2 6 10	2 6 10 14	2 6 10 4	2 6 1 ..	2
94	Pu	2	2 6	2 6 10	2 6 10 14	2 6 10 6	2 6.. ..	2
95	Am	2	2 6	2 6 10	2 6 10 14	2 6 10 7	2 6.. ..	2
96	Cm	2	2 6	2 6 10	2 6 10 14	2 6 10 7	2 6 1 ..	2
97	Bk	2	2 6	2 6 10	2 6 10 14	2 6 10 9*	2 6.. ..	2
98	Cf	2	2 6	2 6 10	2 6 10 14	2 6 10 10	2 6.. ..	2
99	Es	2	2 6	2 6 10	2 6 10 14	2 6 10 11	2 6.. ..	2
100	Fm	2	2 6	2 6 10	2 6 10 14	2 6 10 12	2 6.. ..	2
101	Md	2	2 6	2 6 10	2 6 10 14	2 6 10 13	2 6.. ..	2
102	No	2	2 6	2 6 10	2 6 10 14	2 6 10 14	2 6.. ..	2
103	Lw	2	2 6	2 6 10	2 6 10 14	2 6 10 14	2 6 1 ..	2
104	—	2	2 6	2 6 10	2 6 10 14	2 6 10 14	2 6 2 ..	2

Sons, Inc. Publishers, New York, 1961. R. F. Gould, editor, *Lanthanide—Actinide Chemistry,* Advances in Chemistry Series, No. 71, American Chemical Society, Washington, D.C., 1967: Paper No. 14, Mark Fred, *Electronic Structure of the Actinide Elements.*

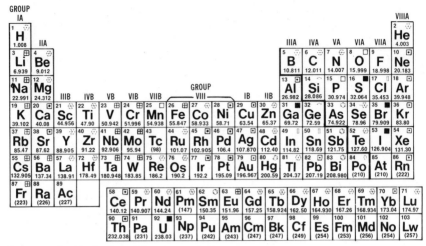

Figure 6.3 Periodic table of the elements.

actual spectra observed, but all the periodic properties of the elements fall into position. Such properties as valence, size, electronegativity, atomic radii for covalent and ionic bonds, ionization potential (which determines whether ionic or covalent compounds will be formed), acid-base character, compound stability, and oxidizing and reducing properties can all be explained by the periodic table thus developed.

An electronic periodic table of the elements is shown in Figure 6.3. Note that the d shell provides the so-called "transition elements" or rare earths, and the f shell makes possible the "inner transition elements" or the actinide series (Table 6.3). The energy levels in Figure 6.2 move closer together in the outer shells of the heavier elements, a characteristic which causes the slight irregularities in properties often noted. The "rare earth" or lanthanide series are all very similar in chemical nature because the external p shell is identical and the internal shells are being filled. Yet the actinide series is close in properties to the corresponding members of the lanthanide series. This similarity was recognized in assigning the names of the actinide elements, most of which were discovered in nuclear research laboratories of the United States (Table 6.3).

THE LAWS OF ABSORPTION

In the laws of absorption of monochromatic radiation by homogeneous transparent systems, the relationship between absorption and thickness was expressed by Bouguer and by Lambert. Each layer of equal thickness absorbs an equal fraction of the light that traverses it. The decrease in radiation over a thickness db is shown by the relationship,

TABLE 6.3 PARALLEL NOMENCLATURE OF THE HIGHER ELEMENTS

Lanthanide Series	Actinide Series
Lanthanum (57)	Actinium (89)
Cerium	Thorium
Praseodymium	Protactinium
Neodymium	Uranium
Promethium	Neptunium
Samarium	Plutonium
Europium	Americium
Gadolinium	Curium
Terbium	Berkelium
Dysprosium	Californium (98)
Holmium	Einsteinium
Erbium	Fermium
Thulium	Mendelevium
Ytterbium	Nobelium
Lutetium	Lawrencium

1.) $$-dI = kI db$$

The effect of concentration on light absorption was expressed by Beer. The fraction of incident light absorbed is proportional to the concentration c of the absorbing material. Beer's law can be expressed as

2.) $$-dI = k'Ic$$

Combining 1.) and 2.) and noting that they show a decrease, we obtain

$$-\frac{dI}{I} = kcdb$$

Integrating I from I_0 to I and b from o to b

$$\int_{I_0}^{I} \left(-\frac{dI}{I}\right) = \int_{o}^{b} kcdb$$

$$(\ln I_0 - \ln I) = kcb$$

$$\ln (I/I_0) = -kcb$$

$$I = I_0 e^{-kcb}$$

In spectrometry the base 10 is used rather than the base e. To convert, we note that

$$\log_{10} (I/I_0) = \frac{\ln_e (I/I_0)}{2.303} = -\frac{k}{2.303} cb = -acb$$

If

$$a = k/2.303$$

Then absorbance = acb, and transmittance = I/I_o. These are standard spectrometric terms.

Absorbance A and transmittance T have the following relationship:

$$-A = \log T, \text{ or}$$

$$A = -\log (I/I_o) = \log I_o/I$$

If two chemical species of different color are present, the absorbance will not be linear with the concentration of one of the species. Hence, the Beer-Lambert-Bouguer law (called Beer's law for brevity) would not apply. If sufficient concentration were present to reduce the light intensity to below the sensitivity of the detector, Beer's law would not apply. If the incident light were not monochromatic, Beer's law would not apply. Hence, in performing an analytical procedure using spectrophotometry or one of its variants, it must be shown that Beer's law applies before the accuracy of the results can be attested to.

ULTRAVIOLET AND VISIBLE COLORIMETRY

Colorimetry is a method of analysis in which a colored solution of unknown concentration is compared with a colored solution of known concentration. Comparison may be visual using Nessler tubes or a Duboscq colorimeter, or photoelectric using a photometer for matching color intensity.

Visual colorimeters rely on the human eye to make a color comparison and on the Beer-Lambert law to establish the concentration. The Nessler method consists in placing a fixed volume of the unknown solution in a glass tube, and comparing the intensity of light passing through it with that passing through a series of similar tubes of equal depth, containing known concentrations of the unknown. This is a classic method of analysis of chlorine or ammonia in drinking water, using a reagent to bring out the color. Colored glass disks are used as artificial standards in the Hellige comparator. A single standard of known concentration can be viewed through the sides of the glass tubes. The more concentrated color is diluted until the colors match. With equal absorbance,

$$A_1 = ab_1c_1 = A_2 = ab_2c_2$$

and since the tubes are equal in diameter,

$$b_1 = b_2$$

The concentrations must be equal, i.e.,

$$c_1 = c_2$$

The most widely used of all color comparators is the Duboscq colorimeter. Daylight is often the light source for this instrument, although a filter offers a more nearly monochromatic light source. The known solution is placed in one cup and the unknown solution in another. Immersed in the cups are glass rods which may be used to vary the sample length until a color match is observed. Again the Beer-Lambert law provides the model for solution. Since the absorbance is equal ($ab_1c_1 = ab_2c_2$), if c_2 is the known concentration, the unknown concentration c_1 can be obtained from the equation $c_1 = c_2b_2/b_1$. The length of cells b_1 and b_2 can be read from the instrument. Visual matching of colored solutions is precise only when the color intensity is low. To maintain this condition, analyses are ordinarily limited to concentrations of less than 2%.

PHOTOELECTRIC COLORIMETERS

To improve the accuracy of color matching, a photoelectric detector is used instead of the human eye. The light passing through the sample activates a photovoltaic cell which generates a voltage readable on an attached meter. A set of known concentrations of the material is used to obtain a calibration curve, and the unknown sample reading is matched on the curve to find its concentration. Precision of 0.5% is ordinarily obtained by this method.

Photometers of various levels of sophistication in their construction are available. Thus, the photocell, if of the barrier layer type, generates a voltage proportional to the incident light; or it may be a vacuum tube the cathode of which is stimulated by light; or it may be a photomultiplier tube which requires an elaborate power supply but is sensitive to very low levels of radiation. Photometers are usually constructed with simple photovoltaic cells; the more elaborate detectors are saved for spectrophotometers. An arrangement of photocells and sample cuvette to improve accuracy is shown in Figure 6.4.

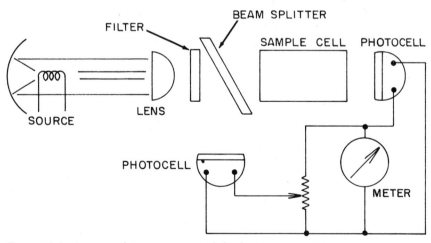

Figure 6.4 Improved arrangement of dual photometer cells.

The figure shows how two barrier layer cells can be employed to compensate for drift in the light source. The radiation passes through a filter (to select the working wavelength region) and then through a beam splitter, which has the property of reflecting a fixed portion of the total light impinging on it. The reflected light is used to standardize the system. The reference photocell is adjusted until the meter reads 100% of scale with only pure solvent in the sample cell. The unknown is placed in the sample cell, and a reading taken of % transmittance. The Beer-Lambert equations are used to calculate the absorbance, and from this the concentration of materials in the sample solution.

SPECTROPHOTOMETERS

A spectrophotometer provides a means for measuring absorption of specific wavelengths by the sample (making it possible to perform an analysis based on a single wavelength), or for performing an analysis based on a fingerprint of absorption at many wavelengths. The first method is a requirement for compliance with Beer's law. The second is a technique for analysis of a complex material, such as an enzyme or protein, which differs little at any given wavelength from similar materials but which can be differentiated if the total spectrum of absorbances is known, i.e., the "fingerprint" method.

The components of the spectrophotometer (Fig. 6.5 A) include a source of continuous radiant energy of appropriate wavelength range; a monochromator, which selects the desired wavelength; a container to hold the sample; a sensor, which responds to the radiation passing through the sample; a photoelectric transducer, which converts the radiation signal to an electrical signal; a secondary transducer, which modifies the signal to make it useful to the display element; and a meter or recorder, which displays the signal.

The source used for production of wavelengths in the visible region from 400 to 800 mμ is a tungsten incandescent lamp. For wavelengths in the ultraviolet region (200 to 400 mμ), a hydrogen lamp is used (Fig. 6.5 B). The source will not be of uniform intensity; hence, to compensate for variation in intensity with wavelength a variable slit is provided. At any given wavelength, the slit is manually adjusted to provide the intensity required. On some instruments, if a variable wavelength scan is made, automatic slit adjustment is available. A double-beam instrument automatically compensates for variations in the source energy.

The monochromator is a combination of components designed to disperse the white light from the source into its component wavelengths, and to pass these wavelengths one at a time through an exit slit to the sample cell. The dispersion may be performed by a prism or by a grating. The resolution between two adjacent wavelengths

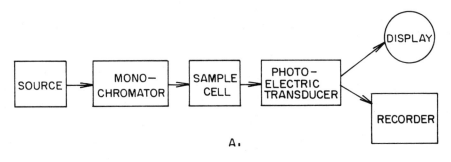

A.

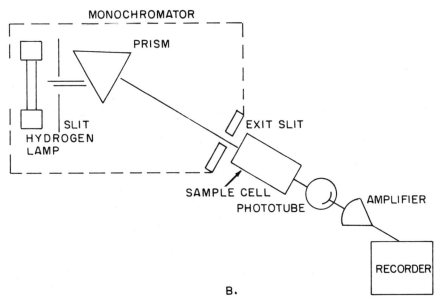

B.

Figure 6.5 Components of a spectrophotometer. *A*, Block diagram; *B*, Typical realization.

varies with frequency in both dispersers; hence, an adjustable exit slit is required to obtain uniform resolution over the band width.

The sample cell in absorption spectrophotometry is of quartz for use in the ultraviolet range, but may be of glass for purely visible analysis. The critical construction detail is the parallelism of the opposite faces.

The phototube is used in the spectrophotometer in preference to the photovoltaic cell. The output of a phototube can be easily amplified, it can be used in the ultraviolet region, and it does not fatigue as does the photocell. The cathode in the phototube is large enough to intercept the entire beam of radiation passing through the sample cell. The impingement of radiation causes a current flow in the tube owing to the electrons released by the radiation. The current flow is amplified by the usual high impedance circuit, and the output is displayed

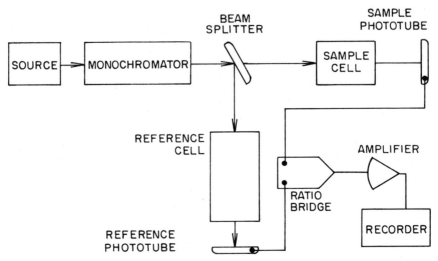

Figure 6.6 Block diagram of double-beam spectrophotometer.

on a recorder whose paper moves proportionally to the motion of the prism, so that a correlation of wavelength and output is obtained.

A double-beam spectrophotometer is pictured in Figure 6.6. The radiation emerging from the monochromator is split into two paths, one containing a nonabsorbing liquid, the other the liquid plus the sample. The beams emerging from the two cells activate two photo-tubes, and the ratio between the transmissions is recorded.

CONTINUOUS PHOTOMETERS

Analysis instrumentation is a term used by the Instrument Society of America to describe instrumentation that has been modified for con-tinuous process analysis. Ultraviolet and visible photometers have been modified for such applications, and some manufacturers specialize in this type of instrument. Considine and Siggia have pro-vided reference works describing instruments used in this applica-tion. Requirements for an instrument of this type have been described by Weiss. The instrumental requirements for a process analyzer that is designed for continuous monitoring of biomedical phenomena at the bedside, in the operating room, or in the research laboratory include the following:

1. The instrument must be rugged. One test for such an instrument in the process industry is to drop it a distance of 10 feet. Another test requires that a maintenance man be able to stand on the process analyzer while repairing another instrument behind a panel.

2. The instrument must operate continuously despite environ-mental difficulties including variations in line voltage, an explosive environment, and ambient temperature changes from 0° to 150°F.

3. The instrument must be self-zeroing and self-standardizing. Automatic equipment is provided for periodic checking of the instrument's zero point and for passing a calibration sample and calibrating itself.

4. Normal conditions of drift and instability are not permitted. Such instruments are built with highly stable equipment, photocells, radiation sources, and rugged sample cells, and are sealed against external corrosion but are able to dissipate heat internally generated. The components are selected for durability rather than price.

5. Rapid and repeatable response is required. High-speed elements should be incorporated into the design to respond rapidly to changes in composition of the continuous sample being monitored or in the intermittent samples being passed through the colorimeter.

INFRARED SPECTROMETRY

A study of infrared spectrometry illustrates the changes that have to be made in equipment when the radiant range is changed. The principles outlined in previous sections are applicable here, but the mode of implementation changes with the special requirements of the field. Sources, detectors, and sample handling techniques are different although analogous. The mechanism for absorption of infrared radiation is based on activation of the vibrational and rotational modes of the molecule, rather than on shifts in the electronic spectra. Because all molecules vibrate and rotate, all show absorption in the infrared region. Figure 6.7 is an abbreviated version of an NBS table illustrating the universality of absorption in the infrared range in organic and inorganic molecules. The availability of low-cost, rugged, bench-type infrared analyzers has made this instrument an indispensable tool for organic chemists engaged for example in the synthesis of new compounds.

One of the conclusions that becomes evident from a survey of Figure 6.7 is that a single wavelength is not enough to identify a compound in the infrared region. The need for a spectrum of the whole region is indicated with the ability to identify the "fingerprints" of the various groups, and to reason out the nature of the compound under study. One can readily see the analogy between the analysis of a compound by infrared absorption bands and the solution of a detective story. One has many clues which must be fitted together in a logical hypothesis to identify the compound. The need for accurate instrumental data is paramount; otherwise the deductions, made from incorrect clues, will lead to incorrect solutions of the problem.

INFRARED INSTRUMENTATION

Most infrared instruments scan the spectrum from 2.5 to 15 μ and are double-beam instruments to provide compensation for sources of

Based on evidence compiled by James E. Stewart of Beckman Instruments. This chart shows the vibrational frequency correlation in the far infrared region. Because research is continuing in the far infrared region, this chart is not all-inclusive.

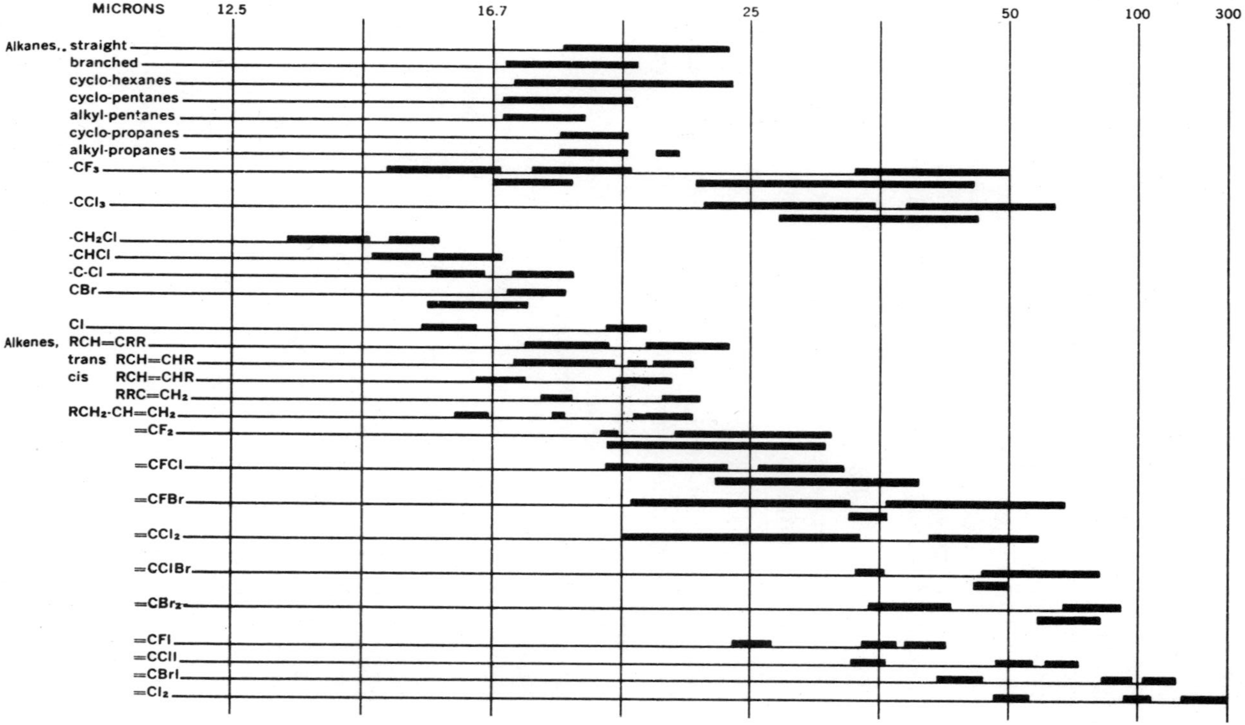

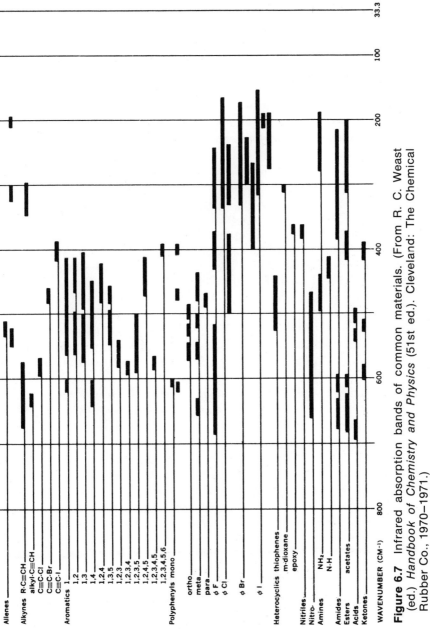

Figure 6.7 Infrared absorption bands of common materials. (From R. C. Weast (ed.) *Handbook of Chemistry and Physics* (51st ed.). Cleveland: The Chemical Rubber Co., 1970–1971.)

drift. Problems can arise in each component of the instrument including the radiation source, the monochromator, the sample holder, and the detector.

To obtain a source of infrared radiation, rich in infrared but low in visible and ultraviolet radiation, two special sources had to be developed, a Nernst glower, or *globar.* Both of these sources are ceramic materials which glow in the infrared region when a current flows through them. The Nernst glower is made of oxides of cerium, zirconium, thorium, and yttrium; the globar is made of silicon carbide.

The monochromator presents a problem, since both glass and quartz absorb in the infrared region. Sodium chloride optics is the rule, although special plastic materials have been developed under the trade name Irtran, which transmit in the infrared. Because of the absorption of infrared radiation by glass and most other materials that can readily be ground optically, mirrors are used instead of lenses, in infrared analyzers. Large crystals of sodium chloride are ground into prisms. But care must be taken to keep moisture away from these hydroscopic crystals. Lithium fluoride, potassium bromide, and calcium fluoride optics are also available, but none of them scans the entire infrared band (1 to 15 μ) in which sodium chloride transmits.

Detectors have to be specially designed for the infrared region. Phototubes and cells are not sensitive to radiation above 1 μ. The heating effect of the infrared radiation is used in the bolometer, which is a coated thermistor. Sensitive thermopiles—fine thermocouple wires hooked in series to amplify the signal—are also used as detectors.

Amplification and recording means are similar to the temperature recorder systems, since we have transduced infrared radiation to temperature at the sensing element. Infrared radiation from the hot ceramic source is split and sent through two paths: one through the sample cell, the other through a reference cell. The beams are positioned so that they alternately pass through a rotating chopper and then through a prism which disperses the beam and scans the wavelength spectrum. Radiation of the selected wavelength is focused by a mirror on the bolometer detector. The amplifier amplifies the AC signal and applies it to the motor which moves the pen, recording transmission as a function of frequency.

CONTINUOUS PROCESS GAS ANALYSIS

The continuous process infrared analyzer was developed during World War II when continuous analysis was important for the manufacture of synthetic rubber. The American version was developed by Pfund at Johns Hopkins University, and the German version by Luft at I.G. Farbenindustrie. These versions are now called respectively the negative filter-type and the positive filter-type infrared analyzer.

They are both non-dispersive, i.e., all regions of infrared radiation are passed through the equipment to the detector. The positive filter-type provides for differentiation of the signal. In the Luft analyzer, both filter differentiation and detector differentiation are provided. Figure 6.8 illustrates both types of analyzer.

In the Pfund analyzer, nichrome wire infrared sources provide a double beam which is chopped by the rotating disk so that only one side is activated at a time. A sample containing the gas to be measured (X) and background gases (Y) is passed through the sample cell. Before arriving at the sample cell, both beams pass through a cell which contains the maximum concentrations of all the gases in the sample except X. Hence, all the infrared patterns characteristic of the back-

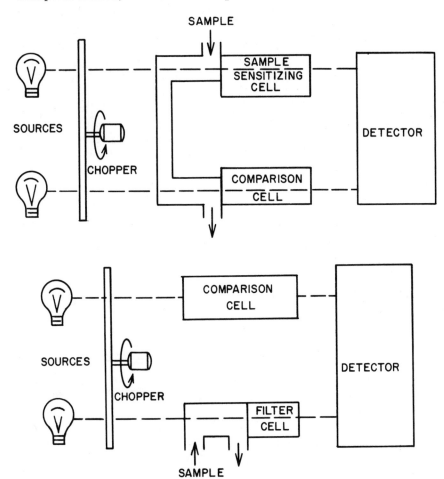

Figure 6.8 Continuous process infrared analyzers. *Top,* Negative filter type; *Bottom,* Positive filter type. (From B. G. Lipták (ed.) *Instrument Engineers' Handbook* (Vol. I). Philadelphia: Chilton, 1969.)

ground will be filtered out in this cell. One of the beams passes through a sample cell containing gas X in its maximum concentration. Emerging from this cell, the radiation beam will possess no infrared spectra characteristic of the unknown gas X. The other beam passes through a cell which contains no infrared absorbing gas (nitrogen, for example); hence, the total absorption of X in the sample will affect this beam. Both beams fall on bolometers sensitive to all wavelengths in the infrared region. The bolometers are combined in a bridge to detect the difference between them as an AC signal, which is amplified, rectified, and recorded.

In the Luft analyzer, one beam of infrared energy passes through the sample cell; the other beam passes through a cell containing Y. All the effects of the absorption of infrared energy characteristic of Y in the sample will be nullified by this reference cell. The detector cell is a gas detector, containing the gas X. When a gas absorbs infrared energy, it increases in temperature and expands. The gas detector then is a detector specific for the gas X. If there were no X in the sample, both gas cells would receive all the infrared energy from the source characteristic of X. The diaphragm between the gas cells would oscillate with equal amplitudes during both halves of the cycle. However, if X is present in the sample, the detector on the sample side of the instrument will receive less energy characteristic of X than that on the other side, the amplitude of vibration of the diaphragm will not be equal, and this difference in amplitude will be amplified by the signal modification equipment to provide a position of the pen on the recorder proportional to the concentration of X in the stream.

These gas analyzers illustrate the ingenuity that can be brought to bear to develop an infrared analyzer for specific applications when circumstances require it.

EMISSION SPECTROMETRY

If a molecule is excited sufficiently by arc, spark, fast-moving particle, or photon, emission spectra are produced. Since the wavelengths found in the emission spectra correspond to the same electrons jumping between the same energy levels as in absorption spectrometry, the wavelength of the emission lines roughly corresponds to the wavelength of the absorption bands. The wavelength lines of the emission spectra are not as obscured by vibration and other artifacts as the absorption spectra; hence, clear separate lines are obtained which are available in tables to eight decimal places. Each element of the periodic table has a unique spectral band by which it can be identified.

Note that infrared absorption spectra have been charted for bonds, not for elements. The C—H bond will have a different infrared spectrum than the C═H bond. Emission spectra are generated when the

C has been split energetically from H, and hence its spectral band is that of C and H independently. The emitted spectrum is analyzed by dispersion into its constituent wavelengths and detected by 1.) the eye in a spectroscope; 2.) a photographic film in a spectrograph; 3.) a photoelectric transducer, and 4.) a display device such as a meter, a digital indicator, a printer, or a recorder. By measuring the wavelength produced, a qualitative analysis is obtained; by measuring the quanta of light emitted by a known sample, a quantitative analysis is obtained.

EXCITATION DEVICES

Unless a spectrograph of the sun or some other luminescent body is being sought, the first problem is to excite the material so that it will emit a spectrum. Devices used for excitation include the flame, the DC and AC arcs, and the spark. The sample is placed in a graphite cup, which constitutes one of the two electrodes. A second graphite electrode of spectroscopically pure material is positioned over the first, so that an arc may be struck between them. Solid metal samples may be machined and used as one of the electrodes. Liquid solutions are placed in the cup or sprayed into the spark gap by an atomizer.

After positioning in the apparatus and properly protecting the operator from the harmful radiation which may result from the excitation, the excitation current is applied. For qualitative analysis, the quantity of energy used in excitation need not be controlled, but for quantitative analysis the same amount of energy must be applied to the arc for each excitation.

The DC arc is the most common method of excitation. A current of 5 to 15 amperes at 220 volts is made to flow through the arc in series with a 10-ohm to 40-ohm resistor. The DC arc has very high sensitivity and is used for low concentrations and for powdered samples. A disadvantage is that the arc may be unstable, as it forms between one spot on the cup and the pointed counterelectrode. The DC arc produces thermal spectra; it operates by heating the sample. If the sample contains volatile components, these will arc first, and thus the spectrum will change with time.

The AC arc is used to eliminate the "hot spot." A discharge of 1000 volts at currents from 0.5 to 5.0 amperes is required. The resistor is connected in series with the arc as in the DC method (to limit the current). The AC arc is useful for the analysis of solutions. The solution is placed in the graphite electrode cup and then heated to remove the solvent. The residue coats the bottom of the cup and is excited by the 60-cycle AC arc.

The high-voltage AC spark produces an exactly reproducible spark voltage. High voltage of 15,000 to 40,000 volts is obtained through a step-up transformer, a capacitor, and a spark generator synchronized with the line voltage. The spark generator is used to ensure that the spark fires only at the moment of peak voltage of the AC source. This form of excitation is best suited to the exact timing of exposures, and it volatilizes only minute amounts of sample. The spark is used extensively in the analysis of metals and alloys.

DISPERSION ELEMENTS

Three types of dispersion elements are used in spectroscopy: prisms, diffraction gratings, and echelles. Since the spectroscope owes much of its success to men like Fraunhofer and Angström, techniques of using prisms have been associated with the names of famous physicists and astronomers.

Newton discovered that a prism will disperse white light into a spectrum of its constituent wavelengths. Light impinging on a prism at a constant angle of incidence i will find itself refracted an angle r according to the wavelength of its constituent parts by Snell's equation:

$$\frac{n}{n'} = \frac{\sin r}{\sin i}$$

where n = refractive index of air
  n' = refractive index of prism material

The simple arrangement for a prism is the Cornu spectroscope. The Cornu prism used in the common spectroscope is constructed of two 30° quartz prisms cemented together. Quartz is birefringent, i.e., it exhibits circular polarization, to prevent which a right-hand polarizing piece of quartz is cemented to a left-hand polarizing prism to produce a 60° prism. Two lenses are required, one to collimate the rays into the prism, the other to focus the rays leaving the prism.

The Littrow mounting uses a single 30° prism with an alumized surface. The light entering the prism is diffracted, reflected, and diffracted again, producing the same effect as the 60° Cornu prism with half the material. Also, the lens which collimates the rays entering the prism also focuses the rays on the return journey. Larger focal lengths are also possible since the length of the equipment is traversed twice by this arrangement.

The dispersion of a spectrograph is measured by the number of angstroms that cover one millimeter on the photographic plate. The dispersion of a prism varies with wavelength. The grating is used because its dispersion is uniform and linear.

As an electromagnetic wave impinges on a grating at an angle of incidence i with grooves of width a, the wave separates into beams at each groove, which may interfere or reinforce each other. The condition of reinforcement is:

$$m\lambda = a(\sin i + \sin r)$$

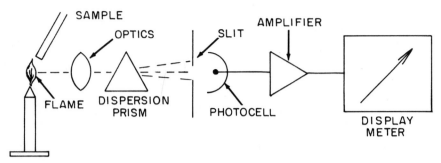

Figure 6.9 Flame photometer.

The angular dispersion with wavelength of the grating would be

$$\frac{dr}{d\lambda} = \frac{\sin i + \sin r}{\lambda \cos r} = \frac{m}{a \cos r}$$

The grating produces multiple spectra because of the integer m, but it is linear with wavelength.

If the diffraction grating is placed on Rowland's circle, no collimating lens is required because of the focusing effect of the grating itself.

FLAME PHOTOMETERS

Another version of spectral analysis is the flame photometer (Fig. 6.9). A solution is sprayed into the flame, and a spectrum is generated which is resolved by an inexpensive prism to a photometric detector. Flame photometry is used for metals, especially for sodium and potassium. Before the flame photometer became available (in 1945), clinical analysis for sodium and potassium by a gravimetric method required several hours of effort. With the flame photometer, the analysis can be completed in about 1 minute.

ATOMIC ABSORPTION SPECTROSCOPY

A combination of flame photometry with the absorption method defines atomic absorption spectroscopy. The atomic spectrum of an element is passed through a flame in which the sample is sprayed (Fig. 6.10). The lines of the element are absorbed quantitatively by the amount of the element in the flame. A single spectrum line is now selected from the resultant radiation and passed into a photometer for measurement. The meter reading from the photometer is an accurate quantitative measure of the concentration of the desired element in the sample.

MASS SPECTROMETRY

Mass spectrometry is an extension of the method of emission spectrometry to ionized particles. A sample is ionized in an electrical

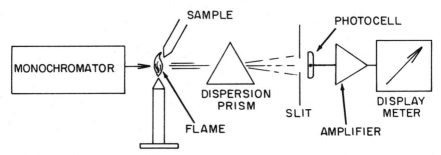

Figure 6.10 Atomic absorption spectrometer.

field and then made to separate in a magnetic field (Fig. 6.11). Each separated mass number is collected and measured by its total ionic charge.

The gas, liquid, or solid sample is introduced into the ionizing equipment at high vacuum (10^{-6} mm. Hg) where it is ionized by electron bombardment, thermal ionization, or spark excitation. The generated ions are accelerated by an e.m.f. to enter the dispersion area.

Methods of mass dispersion utilize passage through a magnetic field, time-of-flight, synchronization of passage through a radiofrequency accelerator, or resonant passage through a quadrupole field.

After separation, the selected ion is accelerated and amplified, and its total charge is either displayed on a cathode ray oscilloscope, an oscillograph, or a chart recorder, or exhibited by a digital display which can be fed into and interpreted by a digital computer.

The mass spectrometer is categorized by the method of dispersion used. The original Dempsey mass spectrometer used a 180° dispersion angle; a smaller unit employing a 60° sector magnetic dispersion is also popular. Other methods of mass dispersion are employed in the magnetic time-of-flight mass spectrometer, the radiofrequency type, and the quadrupole mass spectrometer.

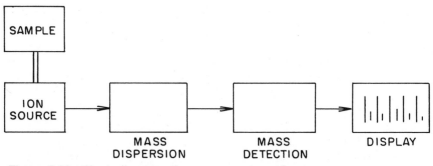

Figure 6.11 Block diagram of a mass spectrometer.

PRINCIPLES OF MASS SPECTROMETRY

Magnetic Dispersion

As the ions are accelerated in the source, their total energy is the original charge times the voltage applied $E = eV$. This energy is the kinetic energy of the moving particle, $E = \frac{1}{2}mv^2$. The dispersion area consists of a magnetic field perpendicular to the direction of motion of the ions in which the force $F = Hev = mv^2/r$ is the magnetic field strength times the charge and velocity; it is also the centrifugal force forcing the particle into a parabolic path. The radius r of the path at any point is

$$r = \frac{(2V)^{1/2}}{H}\left(\frac{m}{e}\right)^{1/2}$$

For any combination of V and H provided by the instrument, a given radius of curvature will be obtained for a given value of m/e. Hence, masses of any m/e ratio can be collected by varying either V, the voltage, or H, the magnetic field of the instrument.

The dispersion angle in mass spectrometers may be either 180°, 90°, or 60°.

Time-of-Flight Mass Spectrometer

In the ordinary mass spectrometer the ions are formed in the ionization chamber and accelerated toward the collector by a series of plates. If the accelerating plates are energized by pulses after ion formation, the ions are accelerated toward the detector with a velocity that is a function of its e/m ratio. Hence, when the ions reach the detector, which is a fixed distance away from the ionizer, they arrive in packets separated by their e/m values. If $e = 1$, the lightest ions arrive first, followed by those with successively higher mass. If an oscilloscope is connected to the detector, a mass spectrum is obtained.

The resolution of the time-of-flight mass spectrometer is limited by the ability of the source to ionize all ions in a sample at the same time. This is a function of the space distribution of the sample and the kinetic energy distribution of the ion gun. Wiley developed an ion gun designed to provide improved resolution by using a double-field source. The first portion of the field ionized the sample and fed it to the second field where the ions were accelerated. A time lag is introduced between the first and second pulses to allow the ionized particles to move into the second region before they are accelerated toward the collector. Features of the resulting instrument include rapid response, high resolution, and simple maintenance.

Connected to the output of a gas chromatograph, this instrument provides identification of each peak by the pattern which appears on the oscilloscope as the peak enters the mass spectrometer.

Radiofrequency Mass Spectrometer

In the radiofrequency spectrometer, the particles are all charged to the same positive energy as they emerge from the ion source. They reach the collector only if their velocity is such that they pass each grid exactly as it reaches the proper negative potential in its cycle. Since the ion velocity is related to the mass number (actually m/e), by varying the frequency, one can vary the mass number of the charged particles that reach the collector.

This instrument has poorer resolution than either the time-of-flight spectrometer or the magnetic instruments, but it is adequate for a lower costing instrument functioning in mass numbers below 100.

Ion Resonant Mass Spectrometer

If perpendicular magnetic and electrostatic fields are applied to a space containing ions, the ions will move through circular paths, which take the form of an expanding spiral. If the electrostatic field is given high-frequency alternation (radiofrequency) at a frequency f, the ion which strikes the collector will have the m/e ratio given by

$$\frac{m}{e} = H/2\pi f$$

The resolution of this instrument varies inversely with the mass number and hence is useful at the low mass number region.

Quadrupole Mass Spectrometer

If four poles are placed as shown in Figure 6.12 and the ionized particles introduced, only one m/e value will traverse the analysis chamber without becoming neutralized by the rods. This m/e value will vary with the acceleration voltage applied. In this spectrometer

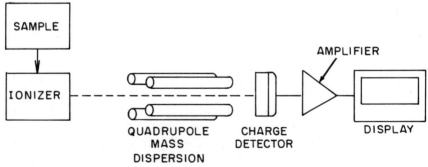

Figure 6.12 Quadrupole mass spectrometer.

the voltage V is scanned linearly, and the various mass numbers appear at the collecting anode as the scan proceeds. The output is displayed on an oscilloscope or light-beam oscillograph.

APPLICATIONS OF MASS SPECTROMETRY

One of the early biomedical applications of mass spectrometry was in the study of respiration. If isotopes of gases are mixed with inspired air and maintained in a closed system with a spirometer, the isotopes can be monitored by the mass spectrometer. These need not be radioactive isotopes which would be required of nuclear instrumentation. The N.A.S.A. and Naval Research Laboratory satellites which analyzed the gases in outer space were equipped with miniature mass spectrometers. Because of the vacuum normally present in outer space, no vacuum system is required for the instrument. The surrounding gas sample continuously passes through the spectrometer. When analysis is desired, the rhenium filament is switched on, the incoming gases are ionized, a permanent magnet is used to disperse the beam, and collectors at positions corresponding to masses of 1, 14, 16, 18, 28, and 32 sense the signals which are amplified and telemetered to earth.

The mass spectrometer has been used for sampling petroleum products, analyzing residual gases, testing for helium gas leaks, and as a detector for gas chromatographs.

X-RAY ANALYSIS

The interest in X-ray analysis is heightened because this range of the frequency spectrum (0.01 to 100 Å in wavelength) is used in analytical methods that extend from absorption and emission to diffraction and fluorescence. Hence, we have an opportunity to review the various techniques available for the interaction of samples with electromagnetic energy. We have pointed out that when another form of energy causes the electrons to jump from one orbit to another, X-ray radiation characteristic of the atom is emitted. When X-rays of the proper wavelength impinge on an atom, they are absorbed and make the electron jump over the same energy path. But in addition to emission and absorption, when X-rays impinge on an atom and cause inner electrons to be ejected, electrons from an outer shell will move into the space, generating secondary X-rays. This process of generating radiation of a frequency different from the impinging frequency is called fluorescence. Another property of X-rays is that their wavelength is small enough so that the atoms in a crystal (spaced on the order of 1 Å apart) appear like a grating to the X-ray and diffract the radiation according to the equation

$$m\lambda = a(\sin i + \sin r)$$

where λ = wavelength
    m = integer multiplier
     i = angle of incidence
     r = angle of refraction
    a = a constant

The other special property of X-rays with which we are all familiar is radiographic. When an X-ray passes through the body, various organs cast different density shadows, making possible the realization of the internal structure by the shadowgraph appearing on a photographic plate.

X-RAY EMISSION

X-radiation is required both for X-ray emission analysis and for the other forms of X-ray analysis based on interaction with the radiation thus produced. There are two forms of X-rays produced; one arises from an electron that passes through an atom. The electron is decelerated, losing energy, and X-ray photons are produced with a frequency of

$$v = (E_i - E_o)/h$$

The electron experiences several such decelerations, and a continuous spectrum (*Bremsstrahlung*) is produced. The other form of X-ray arises when electrons are displaced from inner shells (especially the K shell), and X-ray emission is produced as the energy gaps are filled.

X-rays are generated by Coolidge tubes in which a cathode is heated to generate electrons, which are accelerated to a tungsten target anode, where the Bremsstrahlung effect is produced, which is the continuous X-ray spectrum. The target is turned to focus the radiation on an exit window in the tube, which is made of beryllium.

X-rays are generated for analytical purposes by exciting a sample with a beam of X-rays greater in energy than the characteristic radiation of the sample. The X-ray will penetrate the K region of the atom, and as other electrons drop into the vacated position, secondary radiation will be emitted in the X region characteristic of the material.

Moseley and Bragg provided the fundamental laws of X-ray emission. Moseley postulated that the atomic number of an element is related to its X-ray emission wavelength by the equation:

$$\frac{1}{\text{wavelength}} = KR(Z - s)^2$$

where Z is the atomic number and K, R, and s are constants. To obtain the wavelength spectrum the emission radiation must be diffracted with a crystal according to Bragg's law:

$$n\lambda = 2d \sin \theta$$

where n = order of reflection

d = the spacing between the atoms in the crystal.

The X-ray spectrograph is constructed similarly to the spectrograph for visible light, with the crystal taking the place of the prism or grating, and a Geiger-Müller counter serving as a detector. Instead of the wavelength the angle θ is used as the abscissa in plotting the X-ray spectrum. The spectrum of the unknown material is compared with that of known samples to obtain the analysis. X-ray emission is used mainly for metals, especially in the steel industry.

X-RAY ABSORPTION

The same device may be used for X-ray absorptiometric analysis if an absorption cell is added to the detector. When X-rays are absorbed, two processes occur. Some of the incident energy is converted to exiting X-rays (photoabsorption); the rest is scattered in the sample. The linear absorption is the sum of the photoabsorption and the scattered absorption. Beer's law holds for the total absorption,

$$u = t + s$$

where t = photoelectric absorption coefficient,

s = scattering coefficient, and

$$\frac{I}{I_o} = e^{-udx}$$

where u = absorption coefficient

d = density of material in gm. per cm.^{3}

x = thickness of cell in cm.

e = base of natural logarithms

The absorption coefficient is proportional to the wavelength and the atomic number:

$$\frac{u}{d} = \frac{CNZ^4\lambda^{5/2}}{A}$$

where C = constant

N = Avogadro's number

Z = atomic number

A = atomic weight of absorbing element

The mass absorption coefficient is taken as varying with the cube of the atomic number since A is roughly proportional to Z.

X-ray absorption is useful where the material to be detected is a heavy element such as lead in gasoline or uranium in solution.

X-RAY DETECTORS

Photographic emulsion was the classic material used for detection of X-rays. The difficulty with emulsions is their nonuniformity of response with respect to wavelength, and the time it takes to obtain a good photographic print. Electronic detectors (Geiger-Müller counters) have been brought from the nuclear field and include ionization chambers, scintillation counters, proportional counters, photomultiplier tubes, and cadmium sulfide crystals. The photomultiplier tube used in X-ray absorption analysis is a standard photomultiplier equipped with a phosphor to convert X-radiation to visible light. The Geiger-Müller tube is used in X-ray spectrometry. It is a gas-filled tube with a cylindrical cathode—a single wire anode at 200 to 1500 volts. It discharges when X-radiation ionizes the gas in the tube.

X-RAY DIFFRACTION

When monochromatic X-rays impinge on a crystal, Bragg's law describes the grating effect of the atoms in the crystal:

$$n\lambda = 2d \sin \theta$$

The photographic film detector is preferred for analysis of diffraction patterns, since a 360° photograph is meaningful. Samples for diffraction analysis may be single metal crystals or powder. The goal of the analysis is to define the crystalline pattern. If a single crystal is used and the incident wavelength is known, the spacing of the atoms can be determined by locating a single spot on the 360° field. However, the alignment of the crystal in the holder is often not known. Hence, the rotation of the crystal will produce spots on the circle of film, from which the unit cell size of the crystal can be deduced.

For samples in powder form the Hull-Debye-Scherrer method is used. Since the powder is located in the holder in random orientation, patterns will be detected all around the circle, and each principal diffraction will appear as a circle at an angle 2θ from the incident beam.

X-ray diffraction is useful for the identification of crystalline compounds. Various iron oxides, organic crystalline materials, and minerals in soils can be identified. The X-ray diffraction pattern of approximately 12,000 compounds has been indexed by the American Society for Testing and Materials.

NUCLEAR RADIATION INSTRUMENTATION

Nuclear radiation provides a wide field for the study of biomedical systems. Almost every element can be made radioactive and placed in a biological system so as to trace its performance and function. The heavy elements above bismuth are naturally radioactive and can be used as sources for instrumental methods, for treatment, and for diagnosis. Radiation detection devices have been perfected in the past 30 years or since the beginning of the nuclear age. But we still find the Geiger-Müller counter, the proportional counter, the ionization chamber, and the scintillation counter at the foundation of measurement.

The source of all nuclear radiation is the radioactive disintegration of the nucleus of the heavy elements. The rate of decomposition is always first-order, i.e., proportional to the amount present. For nuclear disintegration of atoms, if N = the number of atoms present,

$$dN/dt = -kN$$

where k = the fraction disintegrating per unit time.

If this is integrated from some initial number of atoms N_0 at some initial time (t = 0) to time t when N = N, then

$$N = N_0 e^{-kt}$$

The half-life is the time $T_{1/2}$ when

$$N = N_0/2, \text{ or}$$
$$\tfrac{1}{2} = e^{-kT_{1/2}}, \text{ or}$$
$$2 = e^{kT_{1/2}}, \text{ and}$$
$$kT_{1/2} = \ln 2 = 0.693, \text{ and}$$
$$T_{1/2} = 0.693/k$$

If we know the half-life we can calculate k, and vice versa.

EMISSION

Emission of radionuclides takes place when the nucleus has an excessive neutron-to-proton ratio. Alpha and beta particles are emitted to increase the charge in the nucleus. After emission of these particles, the internal energy structure of the nucleus becomes rearranged and gamma radiation is emitted. Beta particles are emitted when light elements go through nuclear changes; alpha particles are emitted when heavy elements have radioactive disintegration. Typical nuclear reactions are

$$^{14}_{6}C \rightarrow \ ^{14}_{7}N + \beta^-$$

$$^{226}_{88}Ra \rightarrow \ ^{222}_{86}Rn + \alpha + \gamma$$

The superscript is A, the atomic weight; the subscript is Z, the atomic number. The beta particle is an electron emitted from a neutron in the nucleus, leaving an additional proton. The net effect is to increase the atomic number by 1; atomic weight is not altered. The alpha particle is a helium nucleus and has a weight of 4 and a charge of +2. Its emission reduces the atomic weight by 4 and the atomic number by 2. In the second reaction shown, rearrangement of the energy levels in the nucleus as a result of the alpha emission produces gamma emission.

RADIATION MEASUREMENT

Measurement of radiation requires a knowledge of the range of the three forms of radiation in air and in metal (Table 6.4).

INSTRUMENTATION

Measurement of radioactive particles and waves is by ionization or by scintillation. Alpha, beta, and gamma radiation all produce ion pairs as they pass through matter, i.e., they knock electrons out of atoms, leaving ions behind. A tube filled with gas containing the total ionization produced by an alpha particle need be only several centimeters long; for a beta particle it must be 1 meter long, and for gamma radiation it must be several meters long. Hence, ionization chambers filled with gas are preferred for detection of alpha particles. For beta and gamma radiation, solid ionization detectors (diamond or silver chloride crystals) or semiconductors (germanium and silicon) can be used. High-density metal windows of tantalum or tungsten can also be used in an ionization chamber.

For beta and gamma radiation the scintillation counter is used. A phosphor such as zinc sulfide is made to glow by the passage of the radiation. The glow is detected by a sensitive photomultiplier tube attached to the phosphor.

The ionization chamber can be converted to a proportional counter by increase of the voltage between anode and cathode. When the voltage exceeds 1000 volts, the commencement of ionization in the chamber results in an avalanche. The avalanche, or total ionization of the chamber gas, is used as a count in a modification circuit. Hence, each particle can produce a count, and the number of counts is proportional to the number of particles being emitted during the time of counting.

The Geiger-Müller tube is a counter of the proportional type which contains a material to quench the avalanche. If an avalanche fires and stays fired while several particles enter the tube, only one count will be made. To prevent this, the Geiger-Müller tube contains an alcohol or halogen which suppresses additional ionization in the tube, thus quenching it as the ionization wave hits each quench molecule.

TABLE 6.4 RANGE OF ACTIVITY OF NUCLEAR EMISSION

Form	In Air	In Aluminum
alpha	centimeters	microns
beta	meter	millimeters
gamma	meters	inches

Gas flow proportional counters have open windows; the gas flows directly through the tube, the case of which acts as the cathode. It is used mainly for measurement of alpha radiation, since it permits close contact between the radiation and the detection elements.

Solid-state radiation detectors use semiconductor crystals (either intrinsic or pure, or extrinsic), a thin P-layer on an N-type crystal, or a thin N-layer on a P-type crystal. The nuclear radiation passes through the thin layer and activates electrons and holes at the junction.

SECONDARY RADIATION TRANSDUCERS

Signal modification equipment is required to utilize the very low currents in the ionization chamber (Fig. 6.13) or the pulse generated in the Geiger-Müller counter or proportional counter chamber. Electrometer tubes with very high input impedance are used with the ionization chambers, and specially designed pulse amplifiers are used with the counter-type transducers (Fig. 6.14). The amplified pulses are then counted on an electromechanical counter for slow counts (on an electronic counter for 1000 counts per second, and on a scaler for faster counts). The scaler can be set to count every 10, 100, 1000, 10,000 — and so on — pulses as a single pulse.

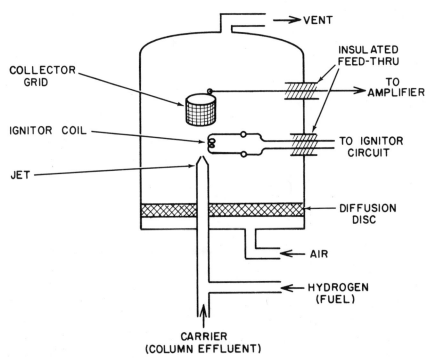

Figure 6.13 Flame ionization detection chamber. (From B. G. Lipták (ed.) *Instrument Engineers' Handbook* (Vol. I). Philadelphia: Chilton, 1969.)

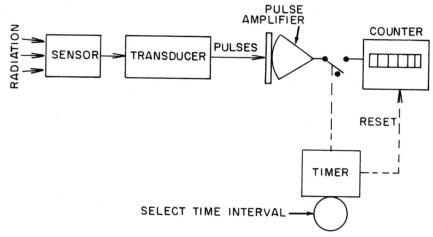

Figure 6.14 Block diagram of radiation counter instrumentation.

The *pulse height analyzer* analyzes the intensity of the pulses and displays statistically how many pulses of each intensity band occur during each counting period. Since different nuclei produce different intensity of pulses, the pulse height analyzer can be used as a spectrum fingerprint device to identify the materials present.

CHROMATOGRAPHIC ANALYSIS

Chromatography, which literally means "colored writing," is the technique of separation of a mixture into its parts by selective adsorption. For example, if a dye is dropped on a piece of blotting paper, it will spread out into bands of different colors, each color representing one of the pure materials in the dye. The Russian botanist, Tswett, assigned the name "chromatography" to the process that he discovered in 1906 for separating the pigment of leaves into its constituent parts. Thus, he found that the red and yellow of fall colors were present in the pigment of the green leaves that he sampled during spring and summer. In his technique, when a suspension of leaf pigment in a beaker was poured into a cylindrical column of calcium carbonate crystals, it separated into bands of color. By breaking the glass, Tswett was able to obtain each separately colored band. Later he found ways of "developing" the column without breaking it by passing pure solvents down the column which dissolved one of the colors.

Tswett expanded the technique to study more than 1000 materials. His body of data was placed on file and not used again until Kuhn and Lederer revived the method in Paris in 1931 for the separation of carotene. Since then, adsorption chromatography has been applied to a range of biological studies. Vitamins, amino acids, nucleic acids, and nucleotides have all been opened to study by this method.

TABLE 6.5 FORMS OF CHROMATOGRAPHY

Mobile Phase	Stationary Phase	Name
liquid	solid	absorption
liquid	liquid	partition
gas	liquid	gas-liquid partition
gas	solid	adsorption
liquid	paper	diffusion
liquid	ion exchanger	ion exchange
liquid	paper–glass	electrochromatography

Liquid chromatography has been expanded from the primitive absorption chromatography just described to partition chromatography, invented by A. J. P. Martin to separate amino acids. The partition method is the basis of paper chromatography, electrochromatography, and gas chromatography.

Chromatography has been defined as a process of differential migration between two phases: a mobile phase and a stationary phase. The mobile phase may be liquid or gaseous; the stationary phase, liquid or solid. Table 6.5 outlines the possibilities.

PARTITION CHROMATOGRAPHY

Partition chromatography is a form of countercurrent extraction. As already stated, the process was invented by A. J. P. Martin for the separation of two amino acids: a water-soluble amino acid and a chloroform-soluble amino acid. The water phase is produced by pouring water on silica gel, where it is absorbed to form the stationary liquid phase. The mobile liquid phase in which the amino acids are suspended (or dissolved in the case of the chloroform-soluble one) is chloroform. As the mixed organic acids move down the column, the water-soluble one is removed first at the top of the column; the chloroform-soluble material remains in the lower portion of the column or is drawn off with the chloroform. As more solvent is added from the top, the bands in the column are developed into different regions in the column. Finally, the bands are eluted or removed from the column by specific solvents. The bands are colorless, but since they are acids, they can be made visible by incorporating an acid-base indicator in the liquid phase of the silica gel.

GAS-SOLID CHROMATOGRAPHY

Gas-solid chromatography is a differential adsorption process. A solid adsorbent in granular form (molecular sieve or activated carbon, for example) is placed in the column. A carrier gas (air or nitrogen) containing a sample of mixed gases like carbon dioxide and methane is passed through the column. The methane is retained longer than the carbon dioxide. Since both gases are colorless, how do we know when they elute from the column? (Elution is performed by additional amounts of carrier gas passing through the column.) A thermal conductivity gas detector is used.

The complete gas analyzer then consists of the components shown in Figure 6.15. An injection port is provided for the injection of sample. The carrier gas continuously flows through the column, and the flow is controlled by the pressure regulator and flow meter. The column, which can be prepared from aluminum, copper, or stainless steel tubing, is filled with the solid adsorbent. The detector is a hot-wire filament or thermistor, whose temperature will vary as the "peaks" of sample are eluted from the column. The temperature of the bead or hot wire affects its resistance, which is measured by a four-legged Wheatstone bridge. The output appears on a meter or, more commonly, on a self-balancing potentiometer.

GAS–LIQUID CHROMATOGRAPHY

In gas-liquid chromatography the solid support is coated with organic solvents, and the gas sample is partitioned on the organic solvent of the column. The apparatus is similar to that shown in Figure 6.15, the only difference being the nature of the material in the column.

Various modifications of gas chromatographs have been developed since gas-liquid partition chromatography first appeared in the United States in 1954. A continuous process chromatograph has been built and marketed. A laboratory version with programmed temperature provides for accurate analysis of mixtures of hydrocarbons con-

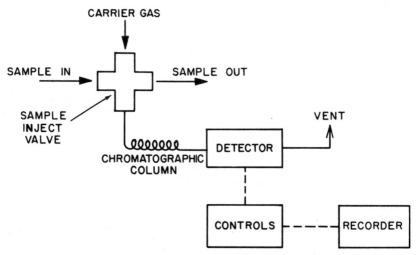

Figure 6.15 Schematic of gas chromatograph. (From B. G. Lipták (ed.) *Instrument Engineers' Handbook* (Vol. I). Philadelphia: Chilton, 1969.)

taining methane with a boiling point of −161.5°C, hexane with a boiling point of 69.0°C, or octane with a boiling point of 125.8°C. Various detectors and detecting schemes have been employed, including flame ionization, electron capture, mass spectrometer, infrared analyzer, and others. The storage of output information to be read out by digital computer has also been carried out.

SUMMARY

Physical methods of analysis have been extensively developed for the past twenty years for the analytical and clinical laboratory and for the process factory. Introduction into on-line patient monitoring and diagnosis is beginning; the topic is discussed in Chapters 8 and 9. The frequency spectrum from DC flow and conductivity analyzers covers impedance methods, audio and ultrasonic methods, radio and microwave frequency methods, infrared, visible and ultraviolet spectrophotometry, and X-ray analysis. In addition we have discussed mass spectrometry, nuclear radiation instrumentation, and various chromatographic analyses.

Ideal spectrometric methods follow the laws of Beer and Bouguer-Lambert. Violation of these laws will produce nonpredictable response, but calibration of the spectrometer in the region of analysis with reference samples is always required for accurate analysis. In every region of the electromagnetic spectrum there is a method of generating a specific type of radiation, a source, a method of placing a sample in the beam, a method of dispersion of the radiation to obtain the wavelengths desired, and a method for detecting these specific wavelengths. The mass spectrometer uses a mass spectrum rather than an electromagnetic spectrum, but otherwise follows a similar schematic of parts, source, dispersion technique, and detection techniques. Chromatographic analysis involves differential migration between two phases as a separation technique. Gas partition chromatography utilizes some of the spectrometric methods as detection systems.

EXERCISES

1. Blood volume can be measured by the isotope dilution method. A 10.0 mg. sample of radioactive isotope with an activity of 4500 counts per minute is injected into the blood. After equilibration, a 100 ml. sample of blood is withdrawn and has an activity of 90 counts per minute, as determined on the same instrument. What is the blood volume of the patient in liters?

2. A respiratory gas sample is subjected to gas chromatographic analysis for analysis of carbon dioxide and oxygen. Four peaks are obtained, of which three are identified. The peaks with their relative integrated areas are given below. Compute the percent composition of carbon dioxide and oxygen in the respiratory gas sample.

Peak	Identity	Relative Area
1	Oxygen	1.5
2	Nitrogen	8.0
3	Carbon Dioxide	0.5
4	Unknown	0.1

3. An unknown sample of biological fluid weighing 10.0 mg. was subjected to infrared analysis. The following relative absorbances were obtained. State whether the fluid contained any of the following materials (by reference to the standard absorption peaks shown in Figure 6.7) and if so, how much? Ethanol, methane, ethane, propane, formaldehyde, benzene, phenol, ether, acetaldehyde, and salts of phosphate, carbonate, chloride, nitrate, and citrate.

Peak	Wavelength, in microns	Relative Area
1	3.00	5
2	3.25	4
3	3.30	1
4	5.5	4
5	6.0	5
6	6.5	2
7	7.0	4
8	7.5	3
9	8.5	4
10	9.0	3
11	11.0	2
12	13.0	1

4. A filter photometer is used to determine red blood cell concentration by comparison with standard samples. The standard sample contains 15 g. of hemoglobin per 100 ml. and produces an absorbance of 0.450. Assuming the samples comply with Beer's law, estimate the hemoglobin content of the following samples:

Sample	1	2	3	4	5
Absorbance	0.895	0.500	0.375	0.250	0.200

General Literature Cited and References

Bauman, R. P. Absorption Spectroscopy. New York: Wiley, 1962.

Dal Nogare, S., and Juvet, R. S. Gas-liquid Chromatography. New York: Wiley, 1962.

Ewing, G. W. Instrumental Methods of Chemical Analysis. New York: McGraw-Hill, 1960.

Harley, J. H., and Wiberley, S. E. Instrumental Analysis. New York: Wiley, 1954.

Hill, N. C. Introduction to Mass Spectrometry. London: Heyden, 1966.

Parker, A., and Rullifsen, S. L. Volatile components in tissue respiration. *Anal. Biochem.*, *19*:418, 1967.

Strobel, H. A. Chemical Instrumentation. Reading, Mass.: Addison-Wesley, 1960.

Wiley, B. N., and McLaren, L. E. Bendix time-of-flight mass spectrometer. *Science 124*, 1956, *Rev. Sci. Insts. 26*, 1150–7, 1955.

Woldring, C. V., Owens, N., and Woolford, J. E. Mass spectrophotometric method for in vivo analysis of partial pressures of gases in blood. *Science 153*:885, 1966.

Chapter 7

Patient Monitoring

NOW THAT we have outlined the principal techniques available for the development of biomedical instrumentation, we shall discuss in detail some of the more prevalent applications. The most rapidly developing applications have been in the field of patient monitoring. Bedside monitoring of critically ill patients has developed rapidly because the sensors were available, secondary amplifiers were readily adaptable, and final display elements were ready for use from data processing applications in industrial and commercial areas. Hence, the engineering fraternity was prepared to supply the technology.

At the same time, medical scientists found that they were using more and more instrumentation to assist in development of advanced medical techniques. We have shown how the physiologist used electronic instrumentation to detect the bioelectrical potentials in the cells and tissues. The molecular biologists made their great breakthrough in understanding the chemistry of DNA, the nucleus, and the cell by use of advanced instrumentation. The surgeon found instrumentation of assistance in advanced surgical techniques, and the physician found electronic equipment useful in patient diagnosis and care.

Hence, in the one place where all these disciplines can converge, the hospital, equipment associated with patient care has developed.

We shall describe the specific sensors used in the hospital for temperature, blood pressure, respiration, and heart rate. The electrocardiogram (ECG) is the center of much of the information logged by continuous instrumentation. A discussion of some common cardiac abnormalities will help to explain how the bedside equipment is used. Details of the electrodes and recorders will illustrate how bedside systems are assembled. We shall then examine the central stations for desired function versus available instrumentation. Next, we shall discuss some of the specific areas of instrumentation used in the catheter laboratory and the operating room.

Hospital instrumentation requirements are such that instruments can be designed in neat little packages that can be connected much as one plugs in the components of a hi-fidelity set—with one exception. If a mistake in plugging in the modules at the bedside is made, the patient may be electrocuted. In addition to incompatibility of electronics, many local hospital situations may create hazards in the use of electrical equipment. Every scientific gain has some limitations. To use the new instrumentation properly, one must be aware of the safety requirements for electrical equipment in general and the safety requirements for electrical equipment in a hospital environment specifically.

SENSORS

The primary variables monitored in patient care units are temperature, blood pressure, respiration rate, and heart rate or pulse.

Temperature is monitored either by a rectal–esophageal probe, or by a surface disk. The sensor is a thermistor encapsulated in a vinyl plastic tip or disk to prevent electrical shorting, and supported by a stainless steel tube (Fig. 7.1). Response time of the probe is about 35 seconds (compared with 3 minutes for a mercury-in-glass thermometer), and its accuracy is ±0.2°F. The standard probe is ³/₁₆-inch in diameter; a smaller probe, 3 mm. in diameter, is available for infants. The tape-on disk for surface temperature monitoring is ³/₈-inch in diameter.

A thermistor is an extremely sensitive temperature transducer which converts a change in temperature to a change in resistance. The active material is a mixture of oxides of manganese, nickel, and cobalt, which is melted and cooled to form an intermediate amorphous–crystalline structure contained in a glass bead. The glass bead is very small and can provide rapid response to temperature. The comparative slowness of response of the medical version is due to the mass of the vinyl tip which provides capacitive lag to the thermal transient.

Because of the amorphous nature of the ceramic material, it has a negative coefficient of resistance with temperature that is approximately logarithmic (Fig. 7.2).

Hence, the resistance-temperature function of the thermistor is nonlinear and has the equation

$$R = R_0 \exp \left(b \left[\frac{1}{T} - \frac{1}{T_0} \right] \right), \text{ and}$$

the expression *exp* is used for raising to a power of e

where T = temperature in °Kelvin at which the resistance is R in ohms, and

T_0 = reference temperature, at which the resistance is R_0 in ohms

The plot of this curve is a negative exponential (Fig. 7.2). For the narrow temperature range of importance to biomedical measurements, i.e., from 68°F to 108°F (20°C to 40°C), the slope is linear within 0.2°F, and hence a direct resistance measurement with an ohmmeter would be accurate. However, when current flows through the thermistor, it is heated, and its temperature is in error owing to this effect. This property of the thermistor is applied to the measurement of respiratory gas flow, and to thermal conductivity detection in gas chromatographs, but in temperature probes the self-heating effect leads to error. The large size (relative to the thermistor) of the vinyl tip on the temperature probe coupled with a limitation of the current flow through the

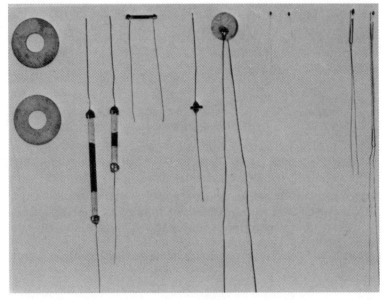

Figure 7.1 Thermistor temperature probes. From left to right: washers, rods(3), discs(2), beads and probes (photo courtesy of Fenwal Electronics, Inc.); resistance sensor: the sensitivity of a thermistor compound and a platinum wire as a function of temperature. Note the small positive temperature coefficient of the platinum and the large negative coefficient of the thermistor. (From S. E. Summer *Electronic Sensing Controls.* Philadelphia: Chilton, 1969.)

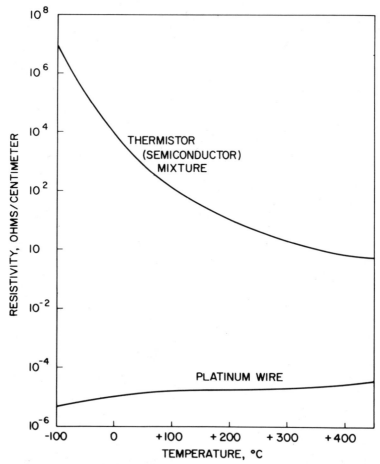

Figure 7.2 Typical temperature-resistance curve for thermistors. (From S. E. Summer *Electronic Sensing Controls.* Philadelphia: Chilton, 1969.)

thermistor is used to maintain accuracy of the temperature measurement. Alternate solutions involve the use of two and four thermistors in a bridge through which the same current flows to compensate for the self-heating effect (Fig. 7.3).

PRESSURE SENSOR

Blood pressure measurement by the sphygmomanometer has been alluded to in previous chapters. The sphygmomanometer utilizes a blood pressure cuff into which air is pumped with a squeeze bulb. The pressure in the cuff is reflected by a mercury manometer or an elastic-element pressure gauge. The sensory element of this system is the physician's ear connected to the sound of the blood in the brachial artery by the stethoscope. Pressure is increased in the cuff until the artery collapses. By means of a valve on the bulb, the physician slowly releases the pressure until sounds heard through the stethoscope (Korotkoff's sounds) indicate turbulent flow has started in the artery. The pressure at which the first sound is heard is called the systolic pressure, corresponding to the peak pressure generated by the heart. The physician continues to reduce the pressure in the cuff until all sounds cease as normal laminar arterial flow returns. At this point he records diastolic pressure, which represents pressure in the artery under relaxed conditions. Obviously, some error is introduced since when the sound ceases, the relaxation has gone beyond that required to match the diastolic pressure of the heart.

Continuous measurement of blood pressure is obtained by inserting a small catheter (sterile hollow fluid-filled tube) into the artery and using a continuous pressure measurement of this fluid stream.

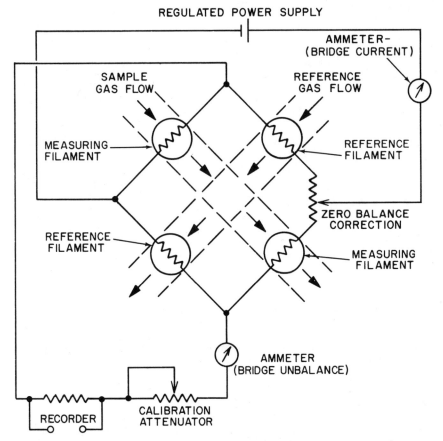

Figure 7.3 Typical circuit for thermistor temperature probe. (From B. G. Lipták (ed.) *Instrument Engineers' Handbook* (Vol. I). Philadelphia: Chilton, 1969.)

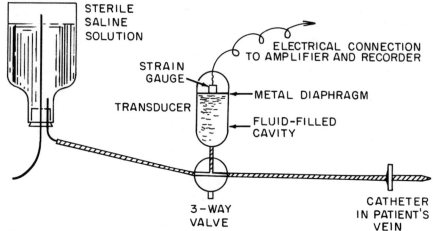

Figure 7.4   Typical arrangement of blood pressure transducer.

The standard blood pressure transducer is a strain gauge mounted on a diaphragm external to the patient, but with a sterile fluid connection to the catheter in the patient's artery. Insertion of a catheter in a vein can be used to monitor continuous venous blood pressure, by use of a second external pressure transducer. The LVDT connection to the elastic diaphragm is also employed. The catheter (Fig. 7.4) is inserted into a vein or an artery. It is filled with a sterile saline solution containing heparin to prevent clotting of the blood. The three-way valve permits 1) filling of the line and the pressure transducer upper chamber with saline fluid, 2) the calibration of the pressure transducer by location of the saline solution a known height above the transducer, and 3) the connection to the catheter for the measurement of blood pressure. The lower portion of the transducer, sealed by the diaphragm from the fluid, contains the strain gauge or LVDT transducer that produces the electrical output which is carried by wires to the monitoring stations at bedside, in the operating room, in the intensive care facility, or in the nurses' central station.

RESPIRATION RATE SENSORS

Respiration rate monitoring is very important in keeping track of the oxygen supply to the vital organs. The expansion and contraction of the chest has been used as a measure of the respiration rate. A belt fastened to the chest with a strain gauge or LVDT transducer attached is used. All sorts of artificial signals (artifacts) may result from random movement of the patient, and since the signal is not recorded directly (which would make it possible for the attendant to observe the artifacts) but is used as an input to a calculating circuit which displays the respiration rate, the artifacts may lead to unreliable readings.

If a heated thermistor is attached to the nose to reflect the change in flow of air, respiration can be detected by amplification and display of the pulse generated. This method is frequently used since the circuitry for detection of thermistor signals is readily available.

New techniques for measuring respiration rate and other respiration parameters by impedance plethysmography will be described in Chapter 8.

HEART-RATE MEASUREMENT

The heart rate as reflected by the pulse rate is an important physiologic measurement in the bedside monitoring of the critically ill patient. It may be derived from the ECG, the technique which will be discussed in the next section, or it may be measured directly. One type of pulse monitor uses a finger strap and attached strain gauge pickup similar to the respiration strap. Another type utilizes the ear oximeter. A small light source and photodiode are attached to the ear lobe. As the color of the blood intensifies with each pulse, light absorption is sensed by the photodiode. The pulse thus formed is amplified so that it may be displayed as the pulse rate.

THE ELECTROCARDIOGRAM

The ECG is the central information source for patient monitoring equipment. From the P-QRS-T wave obtained from chest or limb electrode (see Chapter 4), early information concerning the patient's vital functions is continuously made available. Logic is then built into the data retrieval system to recognize abnormalities in the ECG. The normal ECG has a regular rhythm and a basically unchanging pattern. Electronics can readily detect changes in the rhythm of the wave (cardiac arrhythmias) or missing or premature beats (ectopic foci). More complex (computer) programs would be required to detect car-

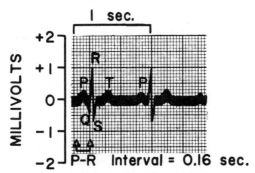

Figure 7.5 Standard electrocardiogram. (From A. C. Guyton *Textbook of Medical Physiology* (3d ed.). Philadelphia: Saunders, 1966.)

diac disease (see Chapter 10). Mechanical activity of the heart produces sounds that can be monitored by phonocardiography (see Chapter 8).

MECHANICAL ACTIVITY OF THE HEART

The mechanical activity of the heart is initiated when the blood from the systemic circulation returns to the right atrium, because the pressure in the veins is greater than the pressure in the atrium. This occurs during the period of diastole, or rest. At the same time, the blood from the lungs returns to the left atrium. The first command given is to the S-A node (represented by the P-wave of the ECG), which orders the atria to contract. During this contraction the atrial pressure increases very little, about 5 mm. Hg, but the blood flows into the ventricles where the pressure increases about 3 mm. Hg. The ventricles are relaxed and yield to the entrance of blood because the A-V node delays the signal to the ventricles.

When the A-V node commands the ventricles to contract, the QRS-complex appears on the ECG. During the early portion of the ventricular contraction, the exit valves of the ventricles are closed, and pressure continues to mount. When the pressure of the left ventricle first exceeds the pressure in the aorta (about 80 mm. Hg), the aortic valve opens.* Rapid ejection of blood into the system occurs, both ventricle and aortic pressures drop, and the inertia of the blood carries it out of the heart and into the circulatory system. The T-wave appears, indicating that the depolarization of the ventricle has started (the wave showing the repolarization of the atrium is concealed in the QRS-complex). The pressure in the aorta and in the lungs is higher than it is in the ventricles, and the exit valves from the ventricles close. These events cause four heart sounds, which can be heard from the surface of the body.

The first heart sound is heard at the termination of atrial contraction when the A-V valves close. The vibration of the valves and of the adjacent walls of the heart causes this sound. The second heart sound occurs at the end of the systole when the aortic and pulmonary valves close. The third and fourth heart sounds occur during diastole. As the A-V valves open and blood flows into the ventricles, the vibration produces a sound. The contraction of the atrium produces the fourth heart sound, which is rarely heard in the normal heart.

A stethoscope can hear only two heart sounds, the first having a frequency of 30 to 100 Hz., the second having a higher frequency (100 to 600 Hz.). There is an interval of about 0.32 seconds between the two audible sounds, then there is an interval of about 0.51 seconds before the next double sound occurs.

---

* A similar process takes place in the right ventricle and in the pulmonary valve.

ELECTRICAL ACTIVITY OF THE HEART

Cardiac electrical activity produces the P-wave, the QRS-wave, and the T-wave at the surface of the body. The first electrical impulse to the atrium is the P-wave, which has a magnitude of 0.2 to 0.3 mv. and a duration of 0.08 seconds. Next comes the QRS-complex, which represents the transmission of the signal to the ventricles, of a duration of 0.08 seconds and exhibiting a maximum height of the R-wave of about 2.5 mv. The final T-wave represents repolarization of the ventricles, with a 0.3 mv. peak and a duration of 0.16 seconds. The standard wave described here is the right arm to the left arm wave, the right arm being connected to the − lead, the left arm to the + lead. The negative wave starts at the right side of the body and moves toward the left.

CARDIAC ABNORMALITIES

To understand the need for signals from the heart, one must understand the form that cardiac abnormalities assume. There are two forms of cardiac malfunction: one involving the cardiac musculature (cardiac myopathies), the second involving the timing of the heart cycle (cardiac arrhythmias).

Abnormal Vectors

The ECG is a one-dimensional representation of a three-dimensional vector. The charge on the surface of the heart represents a dipole, a polarized vector pointing from − to +, the length of which is proportional to the intensity of the potential difference. Most of the analysis of the dipole will work if we assume that the heart is flat and the dipole two-dimensional. For example, let us define the direction from right arm to left arm as positive in the x axis, and the direction from head to toe the y axis. Then the leads I, II, and III provide axes of 0°, 60° and 120° in the clockwise direction (Fig. 7.6 and Table 7.1).* Thus, if as in Figure 7.7 we have a *vector cardiogram* with an R-wave of 1.5 mv. in direction V, we would find an R-wave of 1.2 mv. on lead I, an R-wave of 1.4 mv. on lead II, and an R-wave of 0.2 mv. on lead III, all of which parameters can be obtained by dropping perpendiculars to the three axes. Of course, in practice there is no V, only the three ECG's I, II, and III from which we can deduce V.

The normal electrical axis of the heart is at about 59°, and its angle can be graphically obtained from any two of the lead readings. The vector cardiogram of the heart can be displayed by connecting electrodes from above and below the heart to the vertical plates or to an oscillograph, and electrodes from the left and right sides of the heart

---

* We assume that the limbs do not add to the direction, the point of interest being the site of attachment of the limb to the main trunk.

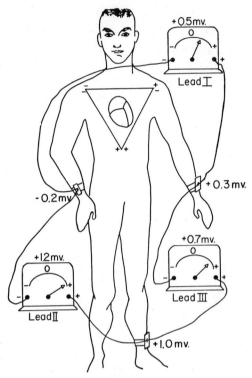

Figure 7.6 Conventional arrangement of electrodes for recording the standard electrocardiographic leads. Einthoven's triangle is superimposed on the chest. (From A. C. Guyton *Textbook of Medical Physiology* (3d ed.). Philadelphia: Saunders, 1966.)

TABLE 7.1 TWELVE STANDARD POSITIONS OF THE ECG LEADS

	Terminal	
	−	+
Lead I	RA	LA
Lead II	RA	LL
Lead III	LA	LL
Chest	Indifferent Electrode	V_1, V_2, V_3, V_4, V_5, V_6
aVF	RA + LA	LL
avR	LA + LL	RA
aVL	RA + LL	LA

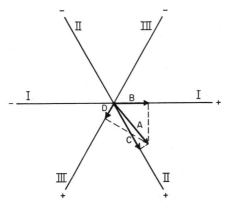

Figure 7.7 Vector cardiograph. (From
A. C. Guyton *Textbook of Medical
Physiology* (3d ed.). Philadelphia:
Saunders, 1966.)

to the horizontal plates. As the vector starts at zero with no activation, moves to its maximum position at 59°, rotates counterclockwise, and decreases to zero, we will obtain the normal vector ECG.

If the heart is hypertrophied, i.e., if the left ventricle is expanded because it has to pump harder against high blood pressure, left axis deviation will be observed. Similarly right axis deviation will occur from right ventricle deviation which may be the result of pulmonary stenosis. Other conditions that can cause abnormal ECG's are listed in Table 7.2.

Cardiac Arrhythmias

Abnormal heart rate may result in a fast rate or tachycardia, or in a slow rate or bradycardia. Tachycardia is caused by increased body

TABLE 7.2 CAUSES OF ABNORMAL VECTOR ECG'S

Left axis Deviation	Right axis Deviation	Remarks
Left ventricle hypertrophy	Right ventricle hypertrophy	Prolonged QRS-
Left bundle branch block	Right bundle branch block	wave
Right muscular destruction	Left muscular destruction	Weak QRS-wave
Decreased QRS voltage	Increased QRS voltage	Remarks
Poor conductivity around heart	Muscle hypertrophy	
Local blocks and diminished muscle		
Fluid in pericardium		
Pulmonary emphysema		

temperature, increased stimulation of the heart by sympathetic nerves, and pathologic conditions like myocarditis (inflammation of heart muscle tissue) and ischemia (obstruction of coronary circulation). Premature beats can be caused by ectopic foci in the heart, which emit abnormal impulses at the wrong time. Ectopic foci result from some form of local irritation, e.g., drugs, nicotine, caffeine, calcified plaques, or local ischemia. Paroxysmal tachycardia is a heart rate that suddenly becomes rapid and then returns to normal, caused by abnormalities in any of the foci in the heart. Atrial fibrillation occurs when many impulses spread from the atrium, arriving at the A-V node at variable periods, causing irregularity in contraction of the ventricle. The ECG shows irregularity of the QRS-complex.

In ventricular fibrillation the ECG is irregular and shows no clear QRS-peaks, the currents in the heart flowing first one way and then another.

ECG ELECTRODES

In continuous hospital monitoring of the ECG, difficulties arise which are not present when a single ECG is recorded. As the patient confined to bed tries to move, the electrodes may be displaced. The electrodes depend on a single conductive spot where conductive paste has been applied with electrolyte to diffuse through the non-conductive layers of skin. As the paste dries, conduction decreases. The paste itself is irritative and may cause a skin reaction. The movement of the patient may provide muscle potentials which obscure otherwise clear ECG readings.

When the ECG is taken in the physician's office, a suction cup with conductive paste is used. The suction cup would wear out quickly in the hospitalized patient confined to bed rest. Instead, a large silver electrode is taped in place; or needle or disk electrodes are used. A biopotential skin electrode is available, made of silver and with a liquid column in contact with the skin.

We have previously pointed out that the impedance registered by the instrument is affected not only by the internal input impedance of the instrument, but by the external impedance of the electrode on the skin. Thus, if the skin electrode impedance is 50,000 ohms and the amplifier input impedance is 50,000 ohms, the amplifier will record only one half the signal, or 1 mv. if a 2-mv. signal is generated. The capacitance between the electrode and the conductive material in the skin produces an RC network which can slow down the response to ECG signals and obscure some peaks.

ECG RECORDERS

The string galvanometer of Einthoven (1903) ushered in the era of clinical electrocardiography. It contains a quartz fiber under tension in a magnetic field, which moves when current passes through it. The string galvanometer was made to intercept a light beam falling on photographic paper, leaving a trace which corresponded to the ECG signal. The quartz fiber was so sensitive that no amplification was required (which was fortunate since amplifiers had not yet been invented). But the impedance of the quartz fiber was so low, that impedance matching was a problem. Electrodes had to be carefully prepared that had low resistance to the skin, otherwise erroneous readings were obtained.

When the voltage generated by the heart is made to pass through a D'Arsonval movement connected to a mirror, a mirror galvanometer is produced. The potentiality of recording the data is obtained by having the light beam impinge on photographic film, a technique that was used for ECG recording in the 1930's.

The standard ECG recorder of the heart specialist uses a heated stylus attached to the D'Arsonval movement. A specially treated waxed paper moves under the heated stylus at a calibrated speed, and the wax is removed by the heat, leaving a dark mark from below the wax as its record. Ink recorders manage to reproduce high frequency records by pressurizing the ink. Frequency response to 80 Hz. is obtained with the heated stylus or an ink recorder. Frequency response to 100 Hz. is obtained by the mirror galvanometer.

For high-speed recording, magnetic tape can be used to store the signal, which can be played back at slower speeds on conventional recorders to show the details.

The Cathode Ray Oscilloscope provides a means for the display of ECG in standard hospital systems. Four to eight channels can be shown on the same oscilloscope by electronically gating each signal in turn, and displaying the scan at a different position on the 'scope.

BEDSIDE MONITORS

The local input in the patient monitoring system is the bedside monitor. Sensor and amplifier are combined to provide a local monitoring station that can be connected into a larger network of individual stations which in turn can be monitored at the nurses' station, a central computer, or some other point.

The sensors described previously are attached to the patient by appropriate electrodes, belts, ear clips, nose clips, and so on, and their transducers convert each sensed variable to an electrical signal. The amplifiers have appropriate input impedances to match the transducers, and proper secondary equipment, such as strain gauge bridges, pulse amplifiers, impedance bridges, and voltage or current amplifiers. The local display provides important information about the nature of the diseases being monitored. Heart patients would have their ECG displayed on a cathode ray oscilloscope. Heart rate, pulse rate, temperature, and blood pressure (arterial, venous, or systemic) would be displayed on appropriate meters. Switches and dials are provided for the physician to set alarm points, i.e., high-level and low-level settings for those variables for which alarms should be sounded. Alarms are ordinarily sounded at the nurses' station; at bedside the alarm appears as a flashing light, visible to the attending nurse but not to the patient. When attention is given to the patient, a switch is thrown, and the flashing light is converted to a steady glow which stays on until the emergency has been attended to.

The recorder is provided for ECG or other emergency data and does not begin to operate until an emergency arises, at which time it is automatically triggered. It can, however, be activated by a manual switch. A selection from various electrodes connected to the patient can be made for display on the recorder.

A cathode ray display tube is useful for many signals, especially the ECG. A tape recorder kept constantly on can provide a running account of the monitoring system; under routine conditions the tape can be erased from time to time. When an emergency arises, however, the tape playback may provide important information concerning the events which precipitated the crisis.

BEDSIDE MONITORING COMBINATIONS

ECG, Pulse, and Heart Rate

The ECG is displayed on an oscilloscope, and the heart rate or pulse rate is selected by throwing a switch below the meter. A visual signal is activated when the heart rate is low or high. The R-wave is determined from the ECG. An ear plethysmograph is attached to determine pulse rate, and the alarm settings and actual rate are shown on the display meter. A three-position lead selector permits selection of the best ECG from the three leads available. A QRS-indicator flashes each time a QRS-complex or pressure pulse is detected.

Systolic—Diastolic Blood Pressure Monitor

The cannula inserted into an artery is connected to a pressure transducer, a carrier amplifier, and a display containing two meters, and shows the systolic and diastolic pressure in mm. Hg. The waveform of the pressure pulse is analyzed by peak selection circuitry to retain the true maximum and minimum pressure, each of which is displayed as the systolic and diastolic pressure. Low and high alarms are available for each meter.

Temperature and Respiration Rate Monitor

Individual panel meters measure temperature in the range 96° to 106°F, and respiration rate in breaths per minute, in the range 0 to 80.

Each meter is equipped with a low and high alarm which can be set by indicators on the meter.

Arrhythmia Monitor

The arrhythmia monitor is used in the Coronary Care Unit for patients who have suffered a myocardial infarction. It is not sufficient to detect fatal arrhythmia, such as occurs in cardiac standstill, heart block, or ventricular fibrillation, it is also necessary to detect ectopic beats, deviation in width of QRS-band, and deviation in rhythm.

The instrument matches continuing ECG patterns with a normal pattern, which can be obtained from the patient and placed in the memory bank of the instrument. The width of the stored normal QRS-wave is compared with each successive QRS-wave. If the width deviates by 0.015 seconds from normal, an ectopic beat is reported. The distance between R-peaks is compared with the normal in the memory bank. If a 20% decrease in the R-R interval is detected, a premature beat is counted.

Most normal ECG's have occasional premature or widened beats; the abnormal condition is indicated when there is a run of widened beats, or an abnormal number of ectopic beats per minute. The instrument computes these data and actuates appropriate signal lights when they occur. Thus, there is a signal light for *run of ectopic beats* and for *frequent ectopic beats,* the former when there are 3 to 6 ectopic beats in succession, the latter when the frequency of ectopic beats is 6 or 12 per minute (selected by the nurse). When muscle signals obscure the ECG, the instrument reacts and actuates an artifact light until the excessive motion by the patient stops and satisfactory ECG's are again received.

RESUSCITATION INSTRUMENTATION

With the knowledge obtained from the development of the instrumentation just described, it now became possible not only to detect the onset of a critical cardiac condition, but also to correct it. The correction is made by medical or paramedical personnel who are called to the patient's side by the bedside monitor alarm, sounded at the nurses' central station, utilizing resuscitation instrumentation that is stationed in the Coronary Care Unit and which can be placed on an emergency cart and rapidly rolled to the bed and set into immediate operation.

The major item on the cart is the defibrillator, connected to large electrodes that can deliver a 400 watt-second pulse for 5 milliseconds—sufficient signal to stop ventricular fibrillation. After this massive shock the heart is completely refractory and may recover its normal rhythm. If it does not, the pacemaker is brought into operation. This device supplies a high-level signal through the chest wall that will stimulate the heart to beat. The signal continues pacing until the heart resumes its own QRS-wave. The pacemaker is designed to provide pulses for either external electrodes or internal connections directly to the heart.

CENTRAL STATION INSTRUMENTATION

The effectiveness of a bedside monitoring station is greatly dependent on the design of the central station console. At the central station, emergency help is available if the attention of the personnel on duty is called to the emergency quickly enough. If a crisis occurs and disappears, a record of it would be helpful for the prescription of subsequent medical care. Meters must be available to register important variables for each patient. A multiple-channel oscilloscope is needed for the display of critical information. A memory unit which will automatically store pre-emergency information would be very useful. A recorder which is automatically switched on during an emergency, or which can be switched on manually by the nurse at any time, is required. The proper selection of audible signals is important. A beeper that provides an audible signal for each QRS-complex for each patient might culminate in meaningless noise if too many patients were simultaneously monitored. Yet an audible buzz calling attention to an emergency will likely initiate useful action.

Hence, the central station must provide an equitable balance of adequate information without audio or visual noise. It must be designed so as to supply the information required without the drawback of collecting useless reams of recorder paper.

Figure 7.8 is a schematic of a central monitoring station; the lower part of the figure represents the instrumentation required at a typical central station console. The cathode ray oscilloscope shown might display 1, 2, 4, or 8 scans. Two to four scans would probably be sufficient to provide information about the four patients being monitored without deluging the nurse on duty with too much data. The switches at the bottom of unit I (on left) allow for selection of the desired ECG or other information.

In the second console shown (Alarm), each little square represents one variable from one patient. Thus, 12 variables from four patients are available. The alarm light will signal high or low, and can be designed with a red flashing light and audible signal when the variable is too high or too low, for example, if blood pressure is too high, or heart rate is too low. The third console is the meter console, on which selected variables from four patients can be monitored. Thus, if a high alarm flashes, this variable can be switched (either automatically or manually) to the meter so that the exact value can be seen. Digital indicators as well as analogue meters are available for this purpose.

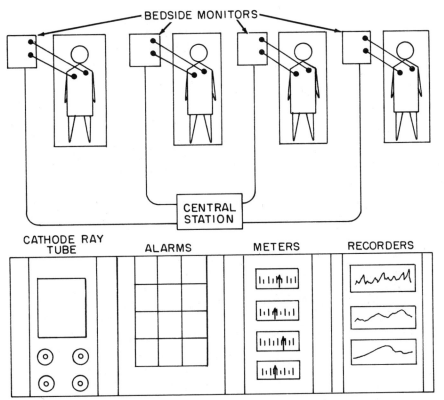

Figure 7.8 Bedside monitors and central station console.

The fourth console is the recording console. If an arrhythmia is detected, the recorder automatically is connected to the ECG. If the pressure pulse is reaching high levels, it can be connected to the recorder. If a heart pacemaker is connected to a patient, the recorder can be connected to follow his heart signals. At the back of the panel, not shown in Figure 7.8, is the control equipment, automatic switches, and memory unit which stores the information for playback on the oscilloscope or the recorder.

The console shown in the figure is an imaginary combination of the useful devices currently available from the manufacturers. In the expanding market new ideas are frequently brought forward. One idea is to send the information to a computer, which can carry out many of the memory functions as well as some of the diagnostic functions that we shall discuss in succeeding chapters. For example, the computer can calculate cardiac or respiratory efficiency from the data provided. The computer can be used to recall on the oscilloscope or the recorder, events that occurred in a previous emergency of the same patient in order to check a diagnosis. The computer can be programmed to calculate the timing of the P, R, and T-waves and compare them with previous normal data in accordance with programmed logic. Thus, just as the analogue arrhthymia monitor can detect arrhythmias and ectopic foci better than the nurse, who cannot watch every ECG of every patient, so the computer can be programmed to watch for symptoms more complex than those used in the arrhythmia monitor.

TELEMETRY

Telemetry is a system which transmits information to a remote point without wires. Thus, physiologic information from astronauts in outer space or on the moon can be transmitted to and recorded on galvanometers on earth. Since this is possible, it seems feasible that medical information from hospitalized patients can be transmitted to a central station in each ward, a central station on each floor, and a central computer in each hospital; and analyzed, recorded, and acted on as required. Patient monitoring in hospitals has expanded so rapidly owing to the availability of the equipment for sensing, modifying, and recording the variables desired. The converse explains the reason for the absence of telemetry in the hospital. The equipment is not yet available in large enough quantities to be useful to the profession. Small numbers of expensive telemetering devices can be provided for the astronauts that cannot yet be provided for hospitalized patients. Many research and development projects are being undertaken, and the extension of telemetry to the hospital may become a reality within the next decade.

SAFETY REQUIREMENTS FOR MEDICAL INSTRUMENTATION

As more sensors, preamplifiers, and recorders are connected to hospitalized patients, the greater are the hazards of electrocution. A healthy person can approach contact with the 110-volt AC line in an electrical outlet, and feeling the tingling in his skin, withdraw before any danger of electrocution occurs; but a patient in a hospital bed attached to electronic gear has no such choice. He is unable to withdraw from the instrumentation firmly attached to his skin. His natural skin resistance has been decreased by the use of electrodes and conductive paste, and in his debilitated condition he has less natural resistance to electrical shock.

The patient in the catheter laboratory or in the operating room, with a catheter in his heart, has less resistance to the surrounding electrical charges. A cardiac catheter connected to an electrical circuit for the measurement of pressure provides a conductive fluid connection directly to the heart. Less than 10 microamperes of current can trigger auricular or ventricular fibrillation, and irreversible fibrillation can lead to death.

Hence, with the expanded use of medical instrumentation to the general public, the responsibility for the proper use of that instrumentation increases. It is, therefore, the reader's responsibility to be aware of both the physiologic implications and the electrical hazards of current flow through the heart and to prevent such current flow by unremitting diligence. Watch for current paths which lead through the heart. Do not compromise with shoddy wiring and old-fashioned plugs in the hospital. Each compromise can cause dangerous accidents and lead to death.

HOSPITAL WIRING PRACTICES

Modern hospitals will be required by the National Electrical Code, Article 517, to isolate general wiring of the hospital from the wiring of the rooms in the critical patient care area. The latter will be isolated electrically from an area in which electrically susceptible patients are treated. The code's definition of an *electrically susceptible patient* is "a patient being treated with a conductor . . . connected to the heart, i.e., the cardiac catheterization area."

However, most hospitals that are already built may not have such isolation areas.

The goal of the code is to prevent a current of even 10 microamperes from flowing through the heart. Since the patient is grounded, any inadvertent source of voltage equal to 5 mv. could produce a current flow of 10 microamperes through 500 ohms of resistance:

$$I = \frac{E}{R} = \frac{5 \times 10^{-3}}{500} = 10 \times 10^{-6} = 10 \text{ microamperes}$$

To prevent this, the maximum potential difference between any two conducting surfaces within reach of the patient, or between either of them and ground, must be less than 5 mv. A patient reference grounding bus is proposed to prevent such exposure.

The patient reference ground bus is a bus wire connected not only to all metal within 5 feet of the patient's bed, but also to the ground connections of all receptacles to which instrumentation used on the patient will be connected. In addition, all the patient reference grounding buses in a room will be connected to a *room ground* (Fig. 7.9). All exposed water pipes and other metal surfaces not normally carrying current will be connected to the room ground. The room ground must be connected by adequate wiring to an appropriate metal structural ground.

These precautions will avert grounding problems, but it will still be possible for an inadvertent failure in an instrument to send a current through the heart to this perfect ground. Hence, isolation from

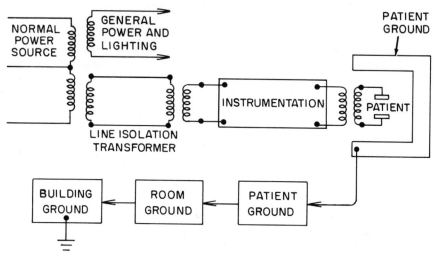

Figure 7.9 Isolation circuits in the hospital.

the instrument is important. Isolation transformers have been suggested as a means of providing this isolation, but they still inductively conduct sufficient current at 60 Hz. frequency to be fatal. Battery operation of patient monitoring equipment would seem to isolate the patient from connection with the major instrument power supply. But again feed through the connector between the sensor circuit and the recorder circuit is possible. The latest proposal is to have an optical link between sensor and amplifier. A battery-operated sensor produces as an output a modulated light signal. The input to the secondary transducer is a photodiode. It is claimed that (A/O Medical Electronics August 1971) adequate precision and frequency response are obtained, and that exposure to leakage current is reduced to below 10 microamperes.

SAFETY HISTORY OF BEDSIDE MONITORS

At this point it will be instructive to review the history of designs of bedside monitoring equipment as related to the shock hazard (Fig. 7.10).

Two-wire System

The first approach was to design bedside monitors as radios are designed, i.e., with one side of the line connected to the chassis (Fig. 7.10 A). One of the patient electrodes is connected to the grid of a tube, a very high impedance point which allows very little current flow. With a two-wire system, the plug could be inserted in its socket backward, placing full-line voltage on the chassis, which is connected directly to the "ground" patient electrode.

Three-wire System

The advent of the three-wire system with a polarized plug reduced the hazard of inadvertently connecting the patient directly to the house current (Fig. 7.10 B). However, there were hospitals in which polarized receptacles were not available, and the third contact was eliminated from the plug to make it fit, which removed the ground completely, and allowed the patient ground to float at some mysterious and hazardous potential. If a fault developed in the instrument circuit, a potential accumulated on the input filter capacitor, which was discharged through the patient, providing an inadvertent defibrillation hazard. A hazard associated with turning the equipment on or off involved the input capacitor — it could be charged to a high potential as it absorbed the transient, subsequently discharging through the patient.

Isolation Transformer

The isolation transformer was the next improvement in safety (Fig. 7.10 C). The input circuit was isolated from the power supply, which in turn could be isolated by a transformer from the patient. However, another hazard emerged which was not obvious to electronics novices — the isolation transformer does not isolate! It does not have infinite resistance at all frequencies. Its impedance is a function of frequency, due to the capacitive reactance between coils, $Z = X_c = 1/wC$, and $I_c = \dfrac{V}{Z} = wCV$. If the transformer capacitance was of the order of 100 microfarads, a current of 3 amperes would flow.

Shielded Transformer

To reduce capacitance between the windings, the configuration shown in Figure 7.10 D was employed. A shield was inserted between the primary and secondary of the input and output transformers in the circuit to reduce capacitive coupling, and the ideal isolation system seemed a reality. Unfortunately, however, it did not prevent accidents. The system was leak proof, but it was not fool proof. An accidental short-circuit somewhere in the system or a malfunctioning vacuum cleaner motor plugged into the same line as the instrument would elevate the ground terminal above ground potential. The current could flow through the patient from the ground to provide shock.

Patient Ground Drive

Another invention was the ground loop detector (Fig. 7.10 E). A meter was connected between the patient leads and ground, and if any current flowed an alarm was sounded. The meter could be set in a configuration in which the patient was nicely isolated, but if a

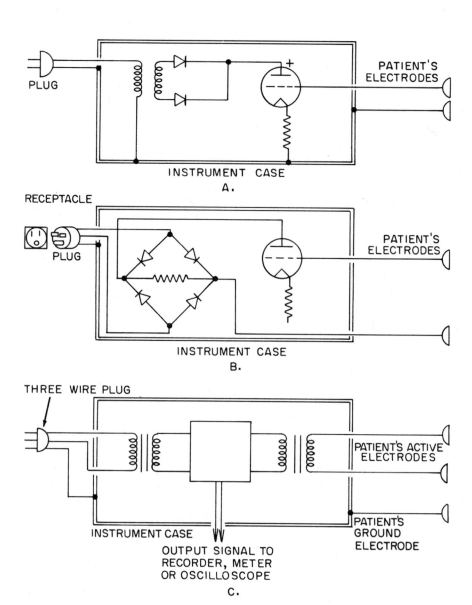

Figure 7.10 Safety history of bedside monitors. *A,* Two-wire system; *B,* Three-wire system; *C,* Three-wire system with isolating transformer; *D,* Shielded transformer; *E,* Separate patient ground drive; *F,* Optical coupling; *G,* Analog isolation system; *H,* Complete isolation by telemetering.

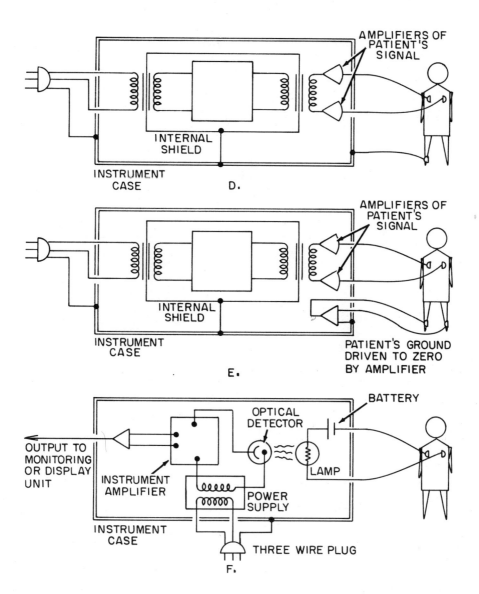

AMPLIFIERS OF
PATIENT'S
SIGNAL

INTERNAL
SHIELD

INSTRUMENT
CASE

D.

AMPLIFIERS OF
PATIENT'S
SIGNAL

INTERNAL
SHIELD

INSTRUMENT
CASE

PATIENT'S GROUND
DRIVEN TO ZERO
BY AMPLIFIER

E.

BATTERY

OPTICAL
DETECTOR

OUTPUT TO
MONITORING
OR DISPLAY
UNIT

INSTRUMENT
AMPLIFIER

LAMP

POWER
SUPPLY

INSTRUMENT
CASE

THREE WIRE PLUG

F.

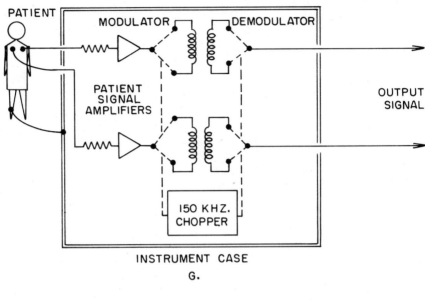

INSTRUMENT CASE

G.

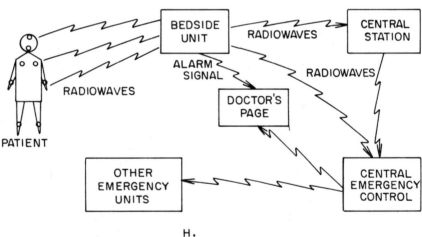

H.

high ground potential closed the meter it would allow 10 milli-amperes of current to flow through the patient, 1000 times that which would trigger fibrillation if it passed through the heart.

Current designs for safety at the time of this writing include the diagrams shown in Figure 7.10 E, F, G, and H. Part E shows a separate patient ground drive (Riggert June 1967 ref H/P 1970). This technique removes the patient–ground connection and replaces it with an operational amplifier in a feedback loop. The patient ground is floating at some safe level which is detected by the amplifier and driven back down to zero level. When the current limitation of the amplifier is exceeded, it ceases to function, but the patient is not connected to ground. Hence, if the patient inadvertently touches a high voltage source, the operating amperage disconnects him from ground, allowing no current to flow through the patient.

Part F illustrates another isolation procedure, optical coupling. The patient is electrically connected with neither hospital line nor ground. A separate battery-operated circuit actuates the electrodes attached to the patient and the output photo source. An electrical transducer is replaced by a phototransducer. The light source reflects the original signal accurately in frequency and magnitude.

The secondary circuit connected to the line has a photodiode input transducer with appropriate frequency, linearity, and amplitude specifications. The patient is completely isolated from external electrical sources and sinks, except for one—every patient is absorbing 60 Hz. radiation from the power lines and other equipment in the hospital. If these pieces of equipment are adequately shielded, there are no objections to this method at this time. The method has had so little field testing at the time of this writing that difficulties in its operation, if in fact there are any, have not yet been detected.

Part G illustrates an analogue isolation system, which partly embodies several of the methods already described. The input signal has a current-limiting resistor and feeds into a floating isolation amplifier, isolated by shielded transformer coupling. The input signal modulates a 150-kHz. signal and is transferred out of the isolation circuit through another intra-winding shielded transformer to the demodulator, which provides a 9-volt to 28-volt DC signal to the display and alarm circuits.

The ultimate solution for the prevention of shock hazards is the telemetering scheme shown in Part H. The combined power supply, sensor, and transmitter are built with microcircuits into the electrode. A separate signal can be sent from each electrode, or a single multiplexed signal can be sent from all the electrodes in each patient. The weak signals can be picked up by the nearby bedside monitor, where the signals can be amplified and sent to the central station. Other emergency signals can be relayed to the physicians' lounge, emergency room, or hospital paging system if emergency aid is needed. Systems like this have been used by N.A.S.A. for retrieval of physiologic data from the astronauts, and are under development for hospital use.

SUMMARY

Patient monitoring equipment in the hospital evolved from research instrumentation used by the physiologist, surgeon, molecular biologist, and diagnostic laboratory technician. Specific sensors are used for temperature, blood pressure, respiration rate, pulse rate, and bioelectrical potentials from the heart. From these data all the patient monitoring signals are collected, processed, and displayed.

The thermistor is the instrument of choice for monitoring temperature. Blood pressure is obtained by transmission of venous or arterial pressure, or both, through a catheter to an external transducer. Respiration rate is obtained from a transducer which responds to the motion of the chest. Pulse rate may be monitored by a finger plethysmograph or ear oximeter. The mechanical activity of the heart is detected by its electrical activity. The QRS-complex of the electrocardiograph activates bedside monitoring equipment for detection of cardiac arrhythmias and other cardiac malfunctions. Special electrodes have been developed for continuous monitoring, and recorders have been replaced with oscilloscopes which display the ECG and alarm devices which record only abnormal periods.

In the bedside monitor, sensor and amplifier are combined to provide the local display required and the source of information needed for other monitoring stations. The local display of meters, indicators, and alarm conditions provides information immediately necessary to establish the patient's condition. Combinations of pieces of equipment are available for different hospital requirements. Resuscitation instrumentation has saved many heart patients when arrhythmia and fibrillation have been detected sufficiently soon to allow for reversal.

Central station instrumentation is effective if all the information required is available, but only information immediately required is displayed. Combinations of alarms, meters, and cathode ray oscilloscope provide the information; recorders and tape memory provide the storage ability for recall or playback. Telemetry systems without wires are not yet perfected, but may be forthcoming within the next decade.

Safety requirements for electronic equipment parallel the side effects of other medical solutions. Care and understanding in dealing with electrical signals is necessary if the use of medical electronics is to be successful. The possibility of microshock from catheters and other electrodes which may take direct paths to the heart must be recognized. Old-fashioned hospital wiring practices do not provide the protection against electrical shock inherent in modern construction. Preventing currents of more than 5 microamperes from arriving accidentally in the leads to an exposed patient is the goal of modern wiring practices. Isolation of instrumentation from the patient by shielded transformers (to prevent inadvertent conduction of high frequencies through the transformer windings) and use of optical isolation practices will tend to ensure the safety of the patient.

EXERCISES

1. Design a bedside monitor and central station, using available units for the survey and control of critical respiratory patients.

2. Hyperbaric chambers are used for operations under high pressure. List the problems involved in using patient monitoring equipment during operations and recovery in high-pressure chambers. Where would you locate the various elements of the system? Design a system for such use.

3. It is proposed to design a transducer for the monitoring of gastrointestinal pressures. Prepare a schematic for such a system and discuss the component you would use for each part.

4. The mercury-in-glass thermometer is fragile, unsanitary, expensive, and wasteful of nursing time. Devise a system for periodic sampling of the temperatures of all hospitalized patients. Describe the components you would use.

5. List the hazards to heart catheterization patients from the catheter and other nearby electrical equipment. How would you ensure safety of the patient? List the precautions you would take and the special equipment you would employ.

6. List the hazards to a patient in an Intensive Care Unit who is connected to bedside monitors and central station. How would you ensure the patient's safety? List the precautions you would take and the special equipment you would employ.

General Literature Cited and References

Bruner, J. M. R. Hazards of electrical apparatus. *Anesthesiology*, 28:2, 1967.

Hewlett-Packard. Using electrically operated equipment safely with the monitored cardiac patient. March, 1970.

Kantrowitz, P. Electric Shock Hazards in the Hospital. Instrumentation Technology, in press.

Medical Electronics. American Optical Corp., Med. Div., Aug., 1971.

Micropower through the heart is a killer. *Design News*, April 1, 1971.

Proposed 1971 National Electrical Code: Vol. 2, 1971 NFPA Technical Committee Reports.

Standards for a Cardiac Catheterization Laboratory. American Heart Assn., 1970.

Chapter 8

Patient Diagnostic Equipment

IN THIS CHAPTER we shall investigate the electroencephalograph, an instrument which records the electrical signals from the brain; the physicians' stethoscope and other instruments of auscultation; the use of ultrasound in medical diagnostics; and instrumental techniques for measuring blood pressure, blood flow, respiratory capacity, and automatic blood analysis. We shall also discuss the impedance plethysmograph, an instrumental technique that may provide nonintrusive measurements for most of the vital functions of the body.

THE ELECTROENCEPHALOGRAPH (EEG)

When electrodes are placed on the scalp, a series of patterns called brain waves are detected. The patterns represent the action potentials of the cerebral cortex—the external surface of the brain—which controls the motor activity of the body, and contains the primary sensory reception areas of the brain. Four types of waves are observed. The primary waves or alpha waves have an intensity of about 50 μv. and a frequency of about 10 pulses per second. Amplification of almost a million times is required to record this signal. The alpha waves appear at the back (occipital) part of the head when the brain is at rest, but not asleep. They normally disappear when the eyes are opened.

Beta waves are detected over the front and midbrain portion of the scalp, and have a lower voltage (5 μv.) and higher frequency (40 to 60 pulses per second) than alpha waves. They seem to appear during tension, or when the patient is exposed to a difficult task.

Delta waves are of very low frequency, less than 4 pulses per second, and are abnormal brain signals; they are found in infancy, conditions of epilepsy, and cerebral tumors.

Theta waves, frequency 4 to 8 pulses per second, appear when the patient is asked to do a task which he cannot perform and consequently seem to be associated with frustration.

The basic rhythms of the brain are outlined in Table 8.1. In general, as the activity of the brain increases, the frequency increases. Thus, the pulses generated during epileptic seizures are of high frequency and intensity, corresponding to the abnormal activity taking place in the brain.

EPILEPSY

Epilepsy, the primary target of EEG studies, may involve either the entire brain, or only a small portion of it.

Generalized epilepsy (entire brain) may be of the grand mal, or petit mal variety. In grand mal epilepsy, neuronal discharges start at one place in the brain, and course through the brain and down the spinal cord to cause convulsions in the entire body. Petit mal epilepsy is localized in occurrence, and may appear in the form of a single muscular jerk, or an isolated period of unconsciousness.

Partial epilepsy encompasses only a localized area, and is associated with a lesion, tumor, or destroyed area of the brain. The seizure produces muscular spasms in the area of the body controlled by the damaged portion of the brain.

The EEG is different for each type of epilepsy, and can indicate the area in the brain where the discharges originate. Removal of these areas has produced remission of symptoms and prevented subsequent attacks.

In addition to the major changes in brain waves symptomatic of epilepsy, and brain damage due to tumors, minor EEG changes have been used to study sleep, depth of anesthesia, and tendency of the individual to suffer a stroke. The brain wave pattern has been correlated with concentration on study, vigilance, or attention to the outside world. Analysis of the EEG has shown when the individual is fatigued and about to make a mistake. Because of the small intensity of brain wave signals, a data-handling technique had to be developed

TABLE 8.1 BASIC RHYTHMS OF THE EEG

Brain Waves	Frequency	Occurrence
Alpha	8–14 per sec.	Awake; quiet; resting
Beta	14–60 per sec.	Tension
Delta	less than 4 per sec.	Deep sleep; infancy; brain disease
Theta	4–8 per sec.	Frustration

to separate the signal from the noise. The technique demonstrates how the proper use of computers and computer algorithms can help in the handling of complex signals.

CORRELATION ANALYSIS

When a periodic component is present in a noisy signal, there are two ways in which the periodicity of the signal can be used to extract it from the noise. The first, autocorrelation, compares the periodic signal with itself repeatedly and accentuates the recurring portion, thus obscuring the random noise. The second method, cross correlation, compares the noisy signal with a clean reference signal with the same period.

The autocorrelation function can be obtained by multiplying F(t), the value of the signal measured at the time t, by its value measured one period later F(t + T), and calculating the average of this product, as

$$\phi(t) = \text{average } (F[t] \cdot F[t + T])$$

It can be seen that this definition can be used in a digital algorithm to have the digital computer calculate the value of $\phi(t)$. Analogue and hybrid computers have also been used to supply the information.

In cross correlation, the second function is a "clean" periodic function of the same period as the signal to be determined, i.e.,

$$\phi_c(T) = \text{average } (F[t] \cdot \sin wt)$$

where $w = 2\pi/T$

CORRELATION ANALYSIS OF BRAIN WAVES

An example of the use of cross correlation is the study of the EEG of a rabbit discussed by Mackay. An EEG transmitter was mounted in the skull of a rabbit, and the pulses detected were recorded on a multichannel instrument. The first channel represented the EEG of the rabbit; the second channel showed a square wave, the rising edge of which represented the illumination of a light in the chamber with the rabbit. Visual comparison of these two signals indicated no apparent correlation. Sending the signals to a computer and performing cross correlation analysis on them produced a definite "evoked response" in the brain wave to the flashing light.

Many more useful experimental results have been obtained by correlation analysis of EEG evoked response to a flashing light. At the University of Missouri (Lago, 1970), 55 male faculty members aged 50 to 60, who had been subjected to a U.S. Public Health Service screening examination for tendency to coronary attack, were given the EEG evoked response test. It was found that two types of evoked response were possible—passive response and active response. Passive response was evoked when the subject merely sat and observed the flashing light. Active response was evoked when the subject was required to perform a task when the light flashed, such as pressing a button to indicate the orientation of a triangle.

The data obtained after 1) performing a correlation analysis in the EEG evoked response to obtain intensity of response; 2) separating the individuals into groups related to their evoked responses; and 3) obtaining a statistical report from the U.S. Public Health Service on the coronary risk test results of the individuals in these groups showed a relationship between the active evoked response and the tendency to coronary disease of the separate groups.

Other studies have shown correlation of the evoked response with the pathologic changes associated with aging (Birren, 1970), with underachievement in college (Bry, 1967), and with the concentration of an individual on his tasks (Daniel, 1967). Steadman et al. (1970) have performed studies that relate the EEG to the state of development of the brain.

PHONOCARDIOGRAPHY

Just as the electrical characteristics of the heart can reveal disease through the ECG, the mechanical characteristics can indicate disease through the sounds generated. In the classic routine examination of the heart, the physician places the stethoscope in an optimum position on the chest and listens to the heart sounds. The phonocardiograph is an instrument for the detection and recording of heart sounds. Components of a typical instrument system include a sensor, signal conditioner, amplifier and recorder, and are matched by a block diagram of the components used for the phonocardiograph shown in Figure 8.1.

NORMAL HEART SOUNDS

There are four normal heart sounds (see Chapter 4), but only two can be picked up by the stethoscope. The other two are too low in frequency and too small in magnitude to be heard. The first heart sound occurs at the start of systole, when the ventricle contracts, closing the A-V valve, and causing pressure waves to bounce back and forth between the valves and the ventricle wall. The second heart sound occurs as blood rushes into the pulmonary artery and the aorta, and the semilunar valves close. Phonocardiograms made inside the

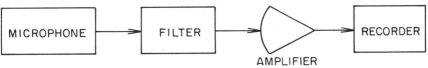

Figure 8.1 Block diagram of phonocardiograph.

heart indicate that the second heart sound occurs in the arteries rather than in the heart. The third heart sound occurs during diastole as the blood rushes into the ventricles. Because the ventricles are relaxed, the sound is very low in frequency. The fourth heart sound is recorded by the phonocardiograph when the atria contract, forcing additional blood into the ventricles.

The areas where the stethoscope is positioned to pick up the two heart sounds are shown in Figure 8.2. As the stethoscope is moved from one area to another, the sounds vary in intensity. The physician is really listening to the functioning of the four valves of the heart, and the optimum audibility is in the vessel into which the fluid has been discharged. Thus, the aortic valve is checked upward in the aorta to the right of the sternum. The pulmonary valve is checked to the left of the sternum, upward along the pulmonary artery. The tricuspid valve is checked at the lower left of the sternum, and the mitral valve is checked where the left ventricle is nearest to the chest, at the apex of the heart.

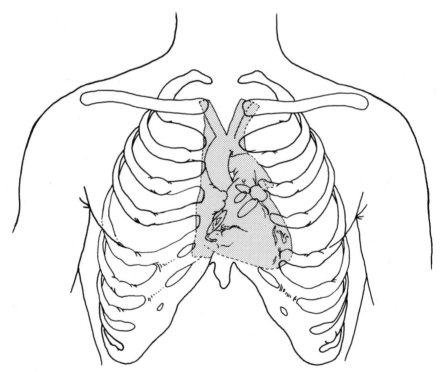

Figure 8.2 Areas for auscultation of heart sounds. (From V. A. McKusick *Cardiovascular Sound in Health and Disease.* Baltimore: Williams & Wilkins, 1958.)

ABNORMAL HEART SOUNDS

Abnormal heart sounds develop from scarring of the heart valves during rheumatic fever of childhood. When the valves become scarred, they may be unable either to open completely (stenosis) or close completely (regurgitation), or both. The sound generated by the valve (murmur) is determined by which of the two conditions predominates. Phonocardiograms of hearts with murmurs readily distinguish between the relative causes. Auscultation provides equally effective detection. The phonocardiogram has been used for mass studies of children to detect the effects of rheumatic lesions, so that early treatment can be started.

Another cause of childhood heart disease is congenital malformation of the heart. The septum between the parts of the heart may not form properly during fetal life, or the left-to-right shunt required when the mother supplies the oxygen for the fetus may not close at parturition. Some of these diseases can be diagnosed by the phonocardiogram; others require additional symptomatic analysis by the physician. Most of the abnormalities can be corrected by cardiac surgery, now that the heart–lung machine is available to provide oxygenation of the blood and to pump the blood through the body during surgical procedures.

Some of the low-frequency heart sounds which are not audible with the stethoscope can be detected by the sense of touch. It is a challenge to the phonocardiograph to provide adequate frequency sensitivity to detect these low frequencies. The technology has provided nomenclature for this difference. Phonocardiography includes detection of sounds from 25 to 2000 cycles; pulse-wave cardiography includes detection from 0.1 cycle to 40 cycles. Both the microphone and the signal conditioner must be designed for the range of use.

DESIGN CRITERIA

In the design of a phonocardiograph system, attention must be devoted to the microphone and to the special signal conditioning required to make the sounds appear like those detected by the stethoscope.

The Microphone

The first phonocardiogram was made by Otto Frank of Munich in 1904. He used a special "segment capsule," a very delicate membrane with very poor frequency response. Einthoven (1907) used the carbon granule microphone. The crystal microphone has been the preferred detection device ever since 1935. The microphone is connected to the body through an air cup. This air volume is equivalent to the air volume in the bell of the stethoscope which absorbs the large amount of low-frequency energy generated by the heart, so that the higher frequencies can be heard, or seen on the recording.

An oscilloscope coupling provides a true picture of all the vibrational frequencies generated. The direct contact microphone is preferred by those who can master the skill of holding it firmly against the skin without producing pressure artifacts. The air-coupled dynamic microphone is also used. The dynamic microphone is similar to a hi-fidelity phonograph pickup, i.e., a fixed magnetic core induces current in the moving phonograph pickup coil as it follows the sound signal. Limited low-frequency response to 150 Hz. is characteristic of this model. The air-coupled crystal can detect frequencies as low as 0.1 Hz., and as high as 2 kHz.

Signal Conditioning

The problem with signal conditioning is, should the signal be conditioned so that the sounds correspond to the bell-stethoscope, or should the signal be conditioned for maximum fidelity? Commercial conditioners provide band-pass filters with 12 decibels (db.) per octave attenuation outside the desired frequency band. Thus, the desired frequency of monitoring can be selected by switching the filter to the following positions:

25 Hz. to 2 kHz.; 50 Hz. to 2 kHz.; 100 Hz. to 2 kHz.; 200 Hz. to 2 kHz.; 400 Hz. to 2 kHz.; and 500 Hz. to 2 kHz.

The decibel unit is widely used in the electronic industry, especially with respect to hi-fidelity equipment. In terms of a voltage signal ratio, the amplitude in db. is 20 log (amplitude ratio)

$$A_{db} = 20 \log A$$

Thus, when $A = 4$

$$A_{db} = 20 \log 4 = 20(0.6) = 12 \text{ db}$$

Hence, a slope of 12 db. per octave reflects a gain of 4. The term *octave* is borrowed from the world of music where it corresponds to a change in frequency (pitch) by a factor of 2.

Commercial phonocardiographs can also be equipped with an automatic gain control, which maintains constant amplitude over the entire spectrum of interest, despite the attenuation of the lower frequencies by the chest and lung cavities.

Recorder Requirements

If signals from 0.1 Hz. to 2000 Hz. are disseminated by the microphone signal conditioning system, the recorder must be able to record them. Unfortunately, light-beam galvanometers have a 3 db. drop at 1000 Hz., and pen-type galvanometers show a drop at 100 Hz.

To compensate for the former condition, commercial instruments provide an amplification in the 500 to 2000 Hz. range of 3 db. per octave, thereby increasing the accuracy of the amplitude recording of the signal by light-beam galvanometers.

APPLICATIONS OF ULTRASOUND

Ultrasound refers to sound waves with a frequency greater than 16,000 cycles per second. These are generated and detected by piezoelectric crystals of barium titanate or other synthetic materials, or by natural piezoelectric crystals of quartz or Rochelle salt. Compression of a piezoelectric crystal generates an electrostatic voltage; application of an electrical field causes the crystal to expand along its piezoelectric axis.

The ultrasonic generator and sensor can be made very small, small enough to be mounted on the head of a cardiac catheter. This ability for "microminiaturization" and the other properties of ultrasonic energy have made ultrasound very popular with the biomedical instrumentation development scientist. Ultrasound can be used instead of X-rays to visualize internal organs. Because of its lower energy, ultrasound can provide a visual profile of soft tissues. Thus, it has been used to locate the midline of the brain, despite the highly absorptive properties of the skull. It is also used to study the heart and liver. Motion can be visualized because of the Doppler effect on ultrasonic signals. We have seen how this effect can be used in the ultrasonic flow meter. Motion of the heart can be visualized by its Doppler effect.

Ultrasonic scanning of the abdominal cavity has provided visual profiles of the fetus in pregnancy, uterine tumors, and the liver and kidneys. The structure of the eye has been examined by ultrasound since 1956, and many eye diseases have been detected by means of it. Ultrasonic scanning has also been used to study the spleen, breast abnormalities, and cervical lumps and nodules.

ULTRASONIC INSTRUMENT SYSTEM

Like every instrumentation package involving radiant energy, the ultrasonic instrument contains a source, a primary modification element, a sample system, a detector, and a display unit (Fig. 8.3). In the case of the ultrasonic instrument, the signal is often generated as a pulse and passed through the biological sample, and the time of passage as well as the output amplitude is noted. To do this there must be coupling between the initial pulse generator and the final display element.

The ultrasonic source is a piezoelectric crystal stimulated by an electrical pulse. The function of the primary modifier in the system is

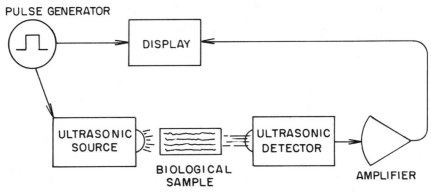

Figure 8.3 Ultrasonic instrument system.

to couple the ultrasonic source to the biological sample with the maximum transfer of ultrasonic energy. The advantage of ultrasound is that it can be focused by a lens just like visible light. The lens may contain a liquid for low absorption of energy (usually water contained in a plastic lens-shaped container).

The pulse now enters the biological material—abdomen, skull, chest cavity, and so on—and is reflected, refracted, and absorbed by the biological interfaces through which it passes. The ultrasonic detector is usually another piezoelectric crystal adjacent to the source, which responds to the reflected energy. Alternate methods of detection include passage through the body with detection on the other side similar to an X-ray, on photographic film. Here, we shall be concerned with the echo-type ultrasonic visualizer.

After detection, the signal is again modified (amplified as an electrical signal) and displayed on an oscilloscope. Three types of display have become standard with the ultrasound graph, namely the A, B, and C scans. The A scan starts when the pulse is generated and continues in time to display the returned scan from the object to be visualized. The B scan has the scope position move geometrically with the probe position on the patient. The C scan produces both x and y coordinates of the probe on the patient, reflected as a two-dimensional display on the oscilloscope. A fourth method of display is the Howry compound scanning, which consists of two motions, one circular and one tangential, of the probe in an attempt to obtain a normal, i.e. perpendicular, reflection from the interface with the organ under study.

Applications

A commercial ultrasonic instrument is provided with several operating frequencies, such as 1, 2.5, 5, and 10 mega-Hz. Frequencies of 1 to 2.5 mega-Hz. are used for intercranial and abdominal regions, and 5 and 10 mega-Hz. for breast and eye probes.

ECHO ENCEPHALOGRAPHY

Echo encephalography is the use of echo ultrasound to visualize the midline of the brain. A brain tumor is often difficult to visualize on X-ray photographs. The echo EEG has proved useful in finding evidence of a tumor which displaces the midline of the brain. An A scan is produced on the memory scope from one side of the brain and then displayed on the same scope displaced in the y direction when viewed from the opposite side of the skull. Careful technique in matching the points diametrically opposite on the skull will produce two scans with identical midline positions in the normal brain, and displaced midline positions if a tumor is present. The equipment is not complex and requires no elaborate scanning table or procedure. It can be used at the bedside of a patient who has had a head injury to detect progressive movement of the midline position (Grossman, 1966).

Holmes (1964) has outlined the result of 12 years' experience in the use of A-scan techniques at the University of Colorado Medical Center, in many applications, such as detecting urine in the bladder without catheterization, measuring the anteroposterior diameter of the liver, and measuring the diameter of the fetal head prior to birth to see if it will move without difficulty through the birth canal.

The visualization of the motion of an interface on the oscilloscope display of the echo ultrasound has been used to study the motion of the mitral valve (Segal, 1966).

In B-scan techniques the transducer is mechanically moved back and forth before the patient, and the resultant echo at each point is shown by a corresponding point on the oscilloscope screen. The B-scan method has generally been replaced by the Howry compound scan (1957), which rotates 110° back and forth around the patient, while traversing a 4-inch vertical path. The patient is immersed in a salt solution which provides contact with the barium titanate transducer. As the transducer moves around the tank, the display on the oscilloscope moves accordingly, visualizing the echo at each point. Instead of immersing the patient in the water, Holmes has built the circular tank with a plastic window against which the patient leans to obtain scans of liver and kidney.

Kohorn has used ultrasonic scanning of the abdomen for the localization of the placenta during gestation (1969). The scan also identifies the location of cervix and lower uterine segment on the basis of internal landmarks. The location of the placenta is very important when intrauterine transfusion is required.

Ultrasonics has proved very useful in the fields of gynecology and obstetrics, replacing X-ray and radioactive procedures which might endanger the unborn child. Proof of pregnancy has been obtained in 8½ to 9 weeks, when the fetal skeleton is not yet visible to X-ray photography. Edema, as well as size of the head of the fetus is detectable; other pathologic findings include collapse of the head when the fetus dies.

The *ophthalmic* surgeon has been using ultrasound both for diagnosis and for treatment (Youdin, 1969); repair of a detached retina without physical penetration of the eye and the liquefaction and removal of vitreous hemorrhage are two of the more dramatic applications of ultrasound.

MEASUREMENT OF CARDIAC FUNCTION

Both blood pressure and blood flow are important diagnostic parameters of cardiac function. Instrumentation for blood pressure described heretofore has been of the invasive type. The physician had to place a catheter in the bloodstream and conduct the pressure through a fluid channel to an external pressure transducer. It is very difficult to perform this invasion each time a diagnostic blood pressure measurement is required, although the procedure is convenient for a bedridden patient who has just undergone surgical treatment or is otherwise disabled because of a critical illness. Hence, instrumental specialists have devoted much time and effort to the search for a noninvasive blood pressure monitor.

Similarly, the rate of blood flow is an important parameter. It is necessary to attach a sensor around a blood vessel to measure blood flow, or blood flow must be deduced from other measurements.

NONINVASIVE BLOOD PRESSURE MEASUREMENTS

One way to measure blood pressure noninvasively is to automate the blood pressure cuff (sphygmomanometer). The procedure (Riva-Rocci) is to attach a cuff around the arm, which is inflated with air by means of a bulb and valve. The blood flowing through the blood vessel (Korotkoff's sounds) is auscultated with a stethoscope. When the cuff is inflated above the systolic pressure, there is no blood flow and no sound. A valve is turned to allow the air to escape slowly from the cuff, and the pressure is measured on an attached mercury manometer. As the blood starts to flow, the sounds of turbulence are heard in the stethoscope; these sounds continue until the diastolic pressure is reached, the blood vessel is held open by the arterial pressure, and laminar flow is obtained. The point at which sound disappears is reported as the diastolic pressure. This technique is automated in the electrical sphygmomanometer.

ELECTRICAL SPHYGMOMANOMETER

A microphone is incorporated in the blood pressure cuff, which is also connected to a pressure transducer. The impulses from the microphone and the pressure transducer are fed to the same amplifier.

The cuff is inflated above the systolic pressure and then slowly re-leased. A recording of the drop in pressure will also reflect the sounds both as the blood begins to flow in the artery, and when diastolic pressure is reached. An automatic pumping and deflation system is used for repeated recording of blood pressure.

ULTRASONIC FLOW METER

If an ultrasonic signal is sent diagonally across a blood vessel, the transit time will be related to the velocity of the blood flow. The experiment is related to the one that Michelson and Morley performed in 1881 in an attempt to determine the velocity of the fictitious ether drift. A source and a detector are mounted as shown in Figure 8.4. With $v = 0$, the time for a signal to move from S to D is $1/c$, where $1 =$ distance from S to D, and c is the velocity of ultrasound in blood. Now if the blood starts to flow, with a velocity v, the effective velocity of the blood in the S-D direction will be $v \cos \theta$; this compares to the previous velocity of ultrasound in blood by the ratio: $\dfrac{v \cos \theta}{c}$. The time of transfer will now be the time with no flow $\dfrac{1}{c}$ times the ratio of velocity change $\dfrac{v \cos \theta}{c}$. The time of transit will then be

$$T = \frac{1v \cos \theta}{c^2}$$

For blood flow through an artery 1 cm. in diameter, the average velocity $= 40$ cm. per second. If the velocity of ultrasound in blood $= 1.5 \times 10^5$ cm. per second, the time $T = \dfrac{1.4 \times 40 \times 0.707}{(1.5 \times 10^5)^2} = 1.8 \times 10^{-9}$ second, a change in 1.8 nanoseconds in the nonflow transit time of 0.1 millisecond. The total measurement is about 0.1% of the signal. A differential measurement can be accomplished by beating the flow signal against a sinusoidal generated signal, and displaying only the beat signal. Although this would undoubtedly cause many problems

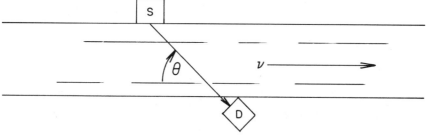

Figure 8.4 Effect of blood flow on signal transit time.

in stability, both electronic and mechanical, these can be circumvented by the Doppler flow meter.

THE DOPPLER EFFECT

When a light or sound wave is reflected by a moving object, there is a change in frequency dependent on the velocity of the object. The Doppler effect is illustrated by the mournful sound of a train whistle augmented by the frequency change in that whistle as it moves away from the depot. In a similar manner, the particles (red blood cells) in the blood reflect an ultrasonic signal, producing a Doppler effect proportional to their velocity:

$$f_r = f_s \sqrt{\frac{c + v}{c - v}}$$

where f_r = frequency received
$\quad f_s$ = frequency sent
$\quad c$ = velocity of ultrasound in blood
$\quad v$ = velocity of blood

Again we have small changes in signal (40 cm. per second) in a large base signal (1.8×10^5 cm. per second), but the method for the detection of modulated frequencies is highly developed in the radiofrequency field.

In operation, two 5 mega-Hz. piezoelectric crystals are used, mounted in a plastic cuff which can be placed around the blood vessel. One of the crystals generates ultrasonic energy; the other, located diametrically opposite the first, detects the energy transmitted by the original crystal as well as the energy reflected from the moving red cells, which is slightly changed in frequency due to the Doppler effect. The beat of the Doppler signal against the original signal produces an amplitude-modulated signal which can be passed into a standard AM radio amplifier to produce a fluctuating voltage proportional to the flow. At a generated frequency of 5 mega-Hz., a shift frequency of 70 Hz. is obtained per cm. per second of flow velocity. This shift frequency can be not only demodulated and recorded but, since it is in the audio region, connected to a speaker and heard.

CARDIAC OUTPUT

The cardiac output–the volume of blood pumped by the left ventricle each minute — is the most important measure of the health of the circulatory system. Hence, much work has been done in the development of methods to determine cardiac output for diagnostic studies. To assist in the understanding of the instruments, we must delve somewhat into the physiology of cardiac output. We shall refer to Dr. Guyton's extensive research in the field (Guyton: Cardiac Output and

Its Regulation, 1963). The normal cardiac output for a healthy adult male is 5.6 liters of blood per minute, but this volume decreases with age, and is 10% less for females. The average cardiac output is 5 liters per minute, but this figure varies considerably with body size. The body surface area of the average 70 kg. human is 1.7 square meters. The cardiac index—the cardiac output per square meter of body surface—approximates 3.0 liters per minute. The cardiac index varies from a value of 4.0 at age 10 to approximately 2.5 at age 80.

For diagnostic purposes, variations from the normal must be related to specific diseases. Thus, there are diseases that cause increased cardiac output, such as beriberi, A-V shunts, hyperthyroidism, and anemia; and there are diseases that cause a decrease in cardiac output, such as myocardial infarction, shock, and severe vascular disease.

Methods of measuring cardiac output are based on the Fick method, employed in the cardiac catheterization laboratory. The patient breathes oxygen from a calibrated container for a standard period of time. A sample of arterial blood is drawn and its oxygen content determined. It is also necessary to determine the oxygen in the venous blood, but this varies with the location of the vein. To obtain a realistic average oxygen concentration of venous blood, the sample is drawn from a catheter in the vein near the right atrium, and the oxygen concentration measured. The cardiac output is determined by the following formula:

$$\text{Cardiac Output} = \frac{O_{2\ IN}}{O_{2\ ABS}}$$

where cardiac output = ml. per minute of blood pumped by the heart

$O_{2\ IN}$ = oxygen consumed per unit time from calibrated container

$O_{2\ ABS}$ = ml. oxygen absorbed per ml. blood = oxygen per ml. in arteries—oxygen per ml. blood in veins

Hence, if a patient consumed 250 ml. of oxygen per minute from the calibrated container, and the arterial oxygen was determined to be 0.20 ml. per ml. blood, and the venous oxygen = 0.15 ml. per ml. blood, the cardiac output would be:

$$\text{Cardiac Output} = \frac{250 \text{ ml. } O_2 \text{ per min.}}{0.20 - 0.15 \text{ ml. } O_2 \text{ per ml. blood}}$$

$$= 5000 \text{ ml. per minute}$$

The dye method avoids catheterization but requires puncture of the artery and a series of samples to be taken for at least 30 seconds. A known concentration of dye (Evans blue) is injected into the cubital vein. A puncture of the artery is made, and small samples are withdrawn and analyzed for the dye. A plot is made of dye concentration per unit time, which consists of a rise to a maximum and a gradual fall. However, before the curve can fall to zero, the dye is being recirculated in the bloodstream. If the falling curve is extrapolated to zero, the time required for the heart to eject all the dye is obtained. If the area under the curve is now divided by this time, an average dye concentration is obtained. The cardiac output is obtained from the following formula:

$$\text{C.O.} = \frac{\text{Dye in}}{\text{Av. con.} \times \text{Time}}$$

where C.O. = cardiac output in ml. per minute
    Dye in = total dye injected in mg.
    Av. con. = average concentration from curve in mg. dye per ml. blood
    Time = time for heart to eject dye in minutes

Thus, if 5 mg. of dye is injected, and the average concentration from the graph is 0.002 mg. dye per ml. blood during an interval of 0.5 minutes, the

cardiac output = 5./0.002 × 0.5 = 5000 ml. per minute

The radioisotope method avoids the arterial puncture, but requires radioactive I^{131} combined with protein to avoid rapid removal from blood. It also requires radiation detection equipment. A record of the radiation in the aorta is obtained by placing a scintillation detector over the aorta and measuring the radiation by means of a rate counter connected to a recorder. One milliliter of the standard isotope solution is injected into the cubital vein, and as it passes through the aorta, a curve similar to the dye dilution curve is obtained. Another milliliter of the same isotope solution is obtained and diluted to a known volume, e.g., 500 ml. After one minute a sample is drawn from the artery. The radioisotope method also allows the total blood volume to be calculated:

$$\text{Blood Volume} = \frac{\text{counts per minute in diluted standard} \times 500}{\text{counts per minute in blood sample}}$$

Since the standard, diluted to 500 ml., provided the numerator, the same standard, diluted by the blood volume, provided the denominator, thus making possible the determination of the blood volume ($\text{Vol.}_1 \times \text{counts}_1 = \text{Vol.}_2 \times \text{counts}_2$). Knowing the total blood volume, we can now calculate the cardiac output:

$$\text{Cardiac Output} = \frac{\text{equilibrium counts} \times \text{blood volume}}{\text{average counts} \times \text{time}}$$

The ballistocardiographic method of estimating cardiac output involves no invasion of veins or arteries. It utilizes Newton's first law ("to every action there is an equal and opposite reaction") to measure the force caused by the ejection of blood from the heart. The patient is placed on a table and carefully suspended so that the pulsatile blood movements are reflected in movements of the table, which are delicately sensed and recorded.

MEASUREMENT OF RESPIRATORY FUNCTION

Quantitative measurement of the efficiency of the breathing function is important for the diagnosis of many respiratory diseases. Obstruction of the airways, lack of compliance of the lung tissue, efficiency of transfer of gases from the alveoli to the blood, and measurement of the tidal volume have valuable diagnostic meaning. Devices have been developed for the measurement of respiration efficiency, ranging from fluorodensitometers to impedance plethysmographs.

The fundamental measuring devices for lung capacity have been the spirometer and the pneumotachygraph. The spirometer consists of a cylindrical bell immersed in water and containing gases that may be inhaled and returned to the bell upon exhalation, where measurements of consumed volume can be made. Some of the measurements made include TIDAL AIR: the volume of a normal exhalation, about 500 ml.; SUPPLEMENTAL AIR: the amount that can be exhaled after a normal exhalation—expiratory reserve volume—about 1600 ml.; COMPLEMENTAL AIR: the amount that can be inhaled after a normal inspiration—inspiratory reserve volume—about 1600 ml.; DEAD SPACE: the amount of inhaled air which does not reach the lungs, but just fills the nasopharynx and the trachea, about 150 ml.; FUNCTIONAL RESIDUAL AIR: the sum of the supplemental and complemental air, about 3200 ml. (functional residual capacity); and RESIDUAL AIR: volume left in the lungs after complete expiration, also known as residual volume, about 1000 ml.

The pneumotachygraph is a device for measuring the flow of air during inspiration and expiration. Plethysmography is the measurement of variations in volume of an organ or a part of the body such as the lungs or thorax. Impedance plethysmography is the use of impedance measurements to detect variations of volume in body organs, such as the size of the heart, lungs, or thorax.

RECORDING SPIROMETER

The displacement of the spirometer can be converted to a recorded signal by any of the techniques described in the section on Sensors, Chapter 3. To secure a proper recording, however, involves proper motivation, stimulation, and careful instruction of the patient.

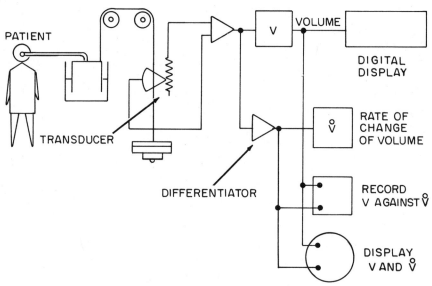

Figure 8.5 Components of instrumented spirometer.

Tidal air volume is obtained by instructing the patient to breath normally. Vital capacity is obtained by requesting the patient to inspire to his maximum capacity and then to expire completely into the spirometer. This measurement is the total of inspiratory reserve, expiratory reserve, and tidal volume. The residual volume, which is the volume of air remaining in the lungs after maximum voluntary expiration, cannot be determined by the spirometer; instead, plethysmography, gas dilution, or nitrogen washout methods are employed.

Other attachments to the spirometer include integrators to display total volumes, derivative units to display rate of inspiration and expiration, timers to produce counts of volume in timed intervals, and digital display elements. A block diagram of an extensively instrumented spirometer is shown in Figure 8.5. An x-y recorder or an oscilloscope provides the compliance measurements required to diagnose the common lung diseases. Early detection and diagnosis of common obstructive pulmonary disease have received a strong impetus from the understanding of the mechanical dynamics of the lung, and from the instrumentation to detect variation in the important parameters of this model.

THE BODY PLETHYSMOGRAPH

The body plethysmograph is a device for measuring the total lung volume, including the inactive residual volume (Fig. 8.6). The patient is enclosed in an airtight box, and his breathing apparatus is connected to a tube from which he can inspire; when he tries to ex-

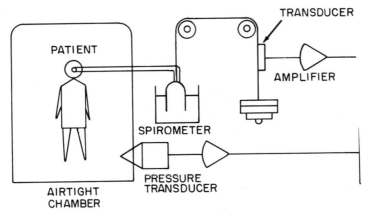

Figure 8.6 Elements of the body plethysmograph.

pire, however, a valve closes, and the total pressure is measured. Upon expiration, Boyle's law applies to the free gases in his lungs excluding the 47 mm. Hg vapor pressure due to moisture. That is, $(P - 47) V = $ constant. Applying this equation to the initial and final pressure and volume:

$$(P_1 - 47)V_1 = (P_2 - 47)V_2$$

If we allow

$$P_2 = P_1 + \Delta P,$$

and

$$V_2 = V_1 + \Delta V,$$

we can solve for V_1 by the following expansion:

$$(P_1 - 47)V_1 = (P_1 + \Delta P - 47)(V_1 + \Delta V)$$

$$(P_1 - 47 - P_1 - \Delta P + 47)V_1 = (P_1 + \Delta P - 47)\Delta V$$

$$V_1 = \frac{(P_1 + \Delta P - 47)}{-\Delta P} \Delta V,$$

which is negative in sign since ΔV must have the opposite sign from ΔP. In the body plethysmograph, P_1 is the initial pressure of the gas in the relaxed lungs; after subject tries to exhale, the pressure increases by ΔP. Now, if there is a value for the initial volume of the lungs, the total volume, V_2, can be calculated. If the vital capacity, measured by the spirometer, is used as the initial volume, the residual volume can be calculated as ΔV.

RESIDUAL GAS ANALYSIS

The functional residual capacity is the sum of the expiratory reserve volume and the residual volume. It is the amount of air remaining in the lungs at the end of normal respiration. If it can be measured, then the residual volume can be determined, since the expiratory reserve volume can be measured by spirometry. The functional residual capacity (FRC) can be measured by the nitrogen wash-out method and other residual gas analyzer techniques.

If at the end of a normal expiration the patient begins to breathe pure oxygen, the nitrogen in his lungs will be diluted by the oxygen and removed in his exhaled air. The total amount of oxygen contained in his exhaled air is a proportion of the total volume of air that was in his lungs at the start of the experiment, the functional residual capacity. Since 78% of the gas in the lungs is nitrogen, the total initial volume,

$$FRC = \text{total volume nitrogen} \times \frac{100}{78}$$

Both residual volume (RV) and total lung capacity (TLC) can be calculated from the FRC, as follows:

$$RV = FRV - ERV \quad \text{and} \quad TLC = IC + FRC$$

where RV = residual volume
FRV = functional residual capacity
ERV = expiratory reserve volume
TLC = total lung capacity
IC = inspiratory capacity
FRC = functional residual capacity

CYBERNETIC DIAGNOSIS OF RESPIRATORY DISEASE

Cybernetics tells us that similar mathematical models can be used for man and machines. One of the ways we can define the functional characteristics of a machine is by step function analysis. A step function is made in the input to the machine, and the resultant output is recorded. By proper mathematical analysis of the output function as a function of the input function, we can define the mathematical characteristics (transfer function) of the machine (Fig. 8.7). This transfer function is also a function of the parameters that define the machine, P_k.

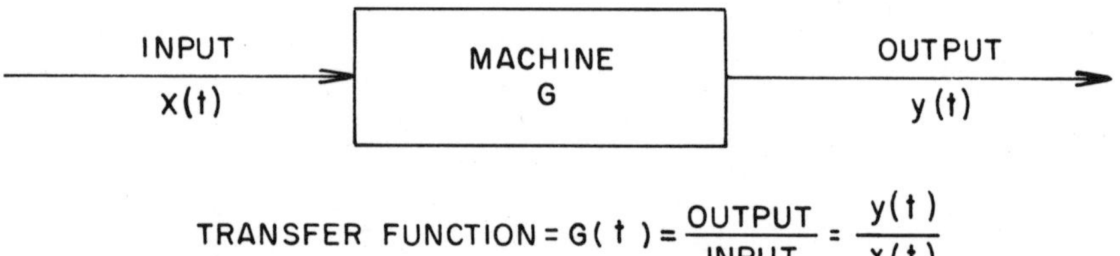

$$\text{TRANSFER FUNCTION} = G(t) = \frac{\text{OUTPUT}}{\text{INPUT}} = \frac{y(t)}{x(t)}$$

Figure 8.7 Transfer function of a machine.

Now, adhering to cybernetic principles, let us replace the inanimate machine by a living organ, e.g., a lung. The input into our lung is a step function called a *pant,* and the patient is taught to perform a step change in air flow rate. The mathematical model of the lung is based on an R-C model of the lung in terms of resistance to air flow and compliance of the tissues. The output of our system is the measured variables obtained from the methods previously described, i.e, the body plethysmograph and the pneumotachygraph.

When the model was developed and applied to actual patients (Feinberg, 1970), differential diagnosis (which agreed with clinical diagnosis) was obtained for patients with emphysema, bronchitis, and asthma (analysis was by a computer algorithm).

SUMMARY

Biomedical instrumentation has been developed for the diagnosis of diseases of the brain, heart, and lungs. Brain waves are monitored by the EEG, which utilizes signals $1/1000$ the size of the ECG. Four types of brain waves are known including alpha, beta, theta, and delta. The alpha and beta are normal waves; the theta and delta result from abnormal conditions in the brain. Epilepsy and brain tumors can be diagnosed and localized. Normal conditions such as sleep and concentration can be studied. Correlation of brain waves with coronary risk is being established by on-going research.

Phonocardiography involves the use of sound and audio electronic equipment to diagnose heart conditions. Of the four normal heart sounds, only two can be detected routinely by the stethoscope. The third and fourth heart sounds are not as interesting from the standpoint of diagnosis as detecting murmurs, which are caused by improper valve formation in the normal heart sound pattern. For population screening for valve malfunctioning, the aortic, pulmonary, mitral, and tricuspid valve functions can be routinely checked by phonocardiography, followed by a medical examination of the subjects with cardiac abnormalities.

Extensive development of ultrasound as a diagnostic tool has resulted from the entrance of the electronic engineer and physicist into the biomedical field. Commercial instruments are available to probe body cavities and the brain with ultrasonic instruments in the regions of 1, 2.5, 5, and 10 mega-Hz. The method is applicable to the midline of the brain, the liver and kidneys, and gynecological, obstetric, and ophthalmic diagnoses.

Diagnosis of cardiac output by modern instrumentation has resulted in development of instruments for the measurement of blood pressure and flow without invasion of the body. Diagnosis of respiratory diseases has inspired instrumentalists to develop automated and instrumented spirometers, pneumotachygraphs, and plethysmographs. The use of cybernetic modeling has been demonstrated for differential diagnosis of lung disease.

EXERCISES

1. The phonocardiogram could be improved if it were indexed to the first and second heart sounds so as to display the areas where the sounds of mitral and tricuspid stenosis and regurgitation appear. Design a data presentation system to accomplish this end.

2. A standard ECG recorder has a cutoff frequency of 100 Hz. What signal-handling equipment could you provide to record a phonocardiograph which has elements of higher frequencies on this standard recorder? Show a block diagram of your proposed system.

3. The EEG shows a time display of the electrical signals from the brain. Much publicity has been given to a machine which records the intensity of alpha activity in the EEG and produces an audible hum proportional to the intensity. Develop a block diagram for a system that would perform this function.

4. Draw a block diagram of the components that would be required to use a Doppler system for measuring the flow of blood in the brachial artery on a noninvasive basis. What modifications would have to be made in your equipment to measure the flow of blood in the aorta?

5. Design a block diagram of a computer system from which cardiac output could be calculated from heart rate and aorta blood flow. Describe sensors that would have to be developed to feed the required information into this program.

General Literature Cited and References

Bates, D. V., and Christie, R. V. Respiratory Function in Disease. Philadelphia: Saunders, 1964.

Birren, J. E. Toward an experimental psychology of aging. Amer. Psychol., 25:124, 1970.

Bry, S. A., Breena, V., and Daniel, L. R. The unresponsive EEG's of college underachievers. Psychonom. Sci., 9:103, 1967.

Butterworth, J. S. Cardiac Auscultation. New York: Grune & Stratton, 1960.

Comroe, J. H., Forster, R. E., Dubois, J. G., and Carlsen, E. The Lung: Clinical Physiology and Pulmonary Function Tests. Chicago: Year Book, 1962.

Daniel, R. S. Alpha and theta EEG in vigilance. Perceptual and Motor Skills, 25:697, 1967.

Dreese, J., and Netsky, M. G. The clinical use of echoencephalography. Virg. Med. Monthly, 90:539, 1963.

Feinberg, B. N., Chester, E. H., and Schoeffler, J. D. Parameter estimation as a diagnostic aid in the determination of obstructive lung disease. Bio. Med. Sci. Inst., 7:55, 1970.

Franklin, D. L., et al. Ultrasonic Doppler shift blood flowmeter. Bio. Med. Sci. Inst., 1: 309, 1963.

Gordon, B. L. (editor) Clinical Cardiopulmonary Physiology. New York: Grune & Stratton, 1960.

Grisham, A. Principles instrumentation and applications of clinical phonocardiography. Measuring for Medicine, Nov. 1966, Feb. 1967, May 1967.

Grossman, C. C. Diagnostic Ultrasound. New York: Plenum, 1966.

Guyton, A. C. Cardiac Output and its Regulation. Philadelphia: Saunders, 1963.

Hewlett-Packard. Heart sound measurement. Appln. Note AN 712, 1969.

Hill, D., and Parr, G. Electroencephalography. New York: Macmillan, 1963.

Holmes, J. H. Medical ultrasonic diagnostic techniques. *Bio. Med. Sci. Inst.*, 2:11, 1964.

Jacobs, J. E. In J. H. U. Brown et al. Biomedical Engineering. Philadelphia, Davis, 1971.

Kohorn, E. I., Campbell, S., and Morrison, J. Placental localization by ultrasonic scanning. Paper 32-4, 8th ICMBE, 1969.

Lago, G. V., and Daniel, R. S. Medical and behavioral correlates of the EEG evoked response in mature adults. *Bio. Med. Sci. Inst.*, 7:75, 1970.

Mackay, R. S. Biomedical Telemetry. New York: Wiley, 1970.

Marshall, R. E., Kooi, K. A., and Ervin, K. H. M. EEG applications of a hybrid electronic correlator. Paper 35-2, 8th ICMBE, 1969.

McKusick, V. A. Cardiovascular Sound in Health and Disease. Baltimore: Williams & Wilkins, 1958.

Nyboer, J., Gessert, W., and Reid, K. A. Counter-force ballistics in man. *Bio. Med. Sci. Inst.*, 4:42, 1968.

Ongley, P. A., Sprague, H. B., Rappaport, M. B., and Nadas, A. S. Heart Sounds and Murmurs. New York: Grune & Stratton, 1960.

Segal, B. L., et al. Echocardiography clinical application in mitral stenosis. *J.A.M.A.*, 195:3, 1966.

Steadman, J. W., Morgan, R. J., and Lambert, P. D. Determination of the developmental stage of the brain. *Bio. Med. Sci. Inst.*, 7:87, 1970.

Suckling, E. E., and Ben-Zvi, S. Formation of images by ultrasonic rays. *Trans. N.Y. Acad. Sci.*, 28, 5:588–595, 1966.

Wichmann, T. F., and Salisbury, P. F. Indirect blood pressure monitoring. *Bio. Med. Sci. Inst.*, 2:185, 1964.

Youdin, M. Application of therapeutic ultrasonic radiation in retinal detachment surgery. Paper 32-6, 8th ICMBE, 1969.

Chapter 9

Advanced Instrumentation and Simple Systems

HAVING DESCRIBED the instrumentation currently in use for bedside monitoring in hospitals and for diagnosis in clinics and physicians' offices, we must now study the instrumentation systems that will be available in coming years. We look to the research laboratory to refine impedance plethysmography—a technique that may become a useful noninvasive diagnostic tool for many diseases. Automating the clinical laboratory will rapidly reduce the number of samples from patients so that test results will be available while the patient is still in the clinic, thus reducing the number of return visits.

Biomedical telemetry should be part of any discussion of biomedical instrumentation. The ability to transmit data without wires leads to many imaginative simplifications of current hospital procedures. For example, the embedment of pacemakers in ambulatory cardiac patients is helping thousands of them survive.

IMPEDANCE PLETHYSMOGRAPHY

Since Nyboer published his data on impedance plethysmography (1959), hundreds of applications to diagnostic and medical measurements have also appeared. Applications to measurement of heart rate and respiration, and nerve and muscular activity; to the function of the endocrine glands and the autonomic nervous system; and to rheoencephalography (REG)—the circulation of the brain—have all been described. During this same period, articles occasionally appeared claiming that the measurements of impedance plethysmography are artifacts, adventitious readings not related to physiologic events.

Analysis of the technique will be aided by reference to the section in Chapter 5 on Conductimetric Measurements and to the section in Chapter 3 on Bridge Circuits. These sections will be very helpful in understanding the concept and development of the impedance plethysmograph, and hopefully will resolve some of the problems associated with it.

MEASUREMENT OF IMPEDANCE

Impedance is a vector quantity, which can be expressed by a complex number,

$$Z = R + \frac{1}{jwC}$$

since

$$j^2 = -1$$

$$Z = R + \left(-\frac{j^2}{jwC}\right) = R - \frac{j}{wC}$$

since

$$Z = R - jX_c$$

Hence,

$$X_c = \frac{1}{wC}$$

The magnitude of $/Z/$

$$/Z/ = \sqrt{R^2 + X_c^2}$$

and the phase angle

$$\phi = \tan^{-1} \frac{X_c}{R}$$

which can be represented geometrically by Figure 9.1. The impedance matching bridge shown in Figure 9.2 is a combination of the bridges previously developed in Chapters 3 and 5 for the measurement of the impedance of biological materials. This configuration is known as the bipolar configuration, only two electrodes being placed in contact with the biological system to be measured.

The prevalent popular impedance measurement device is the tetrapolar impedance bridge (Fig. 9.3).

The impedance of the patient is bucked by inverting the phase of the transformer against the known impedance of the resistance-

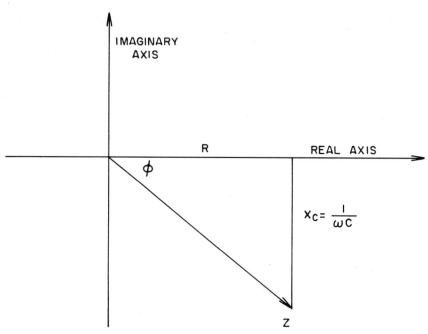

Figure 9.1 Capacitance-resistance-impedance vector.

capacitance (RC) tuned circuit. By setting the reference RC to the baseline level of the patient's impedance, changes appear on the detector. Electrodes 1 and 2 are the source electrodes, and 3 and 4 are the detector or measuring electrodes. By evolution, 100 kHz. has been used as the frequency of operation, although, as we shall see, other frequencies are used for specific measurements. Note the patient isolation provided by the transformer connections to the electrodes, which would not be effective if a common chassis ground were used.

A modification of the Nyboer bridge is shown in Figure 9.4. Operational amplifiers are used to obtain constant current across the patient circuit in order to nullify the impedances of electrodes 1 and 2, and a high impedance operational amplifier circuit is used to nullify the impedances of electrodes 3 and 4.

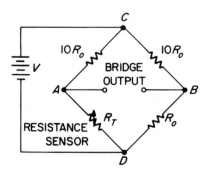

Figure 9.2 Impedance matching bridge. (From S. E. Summer *Electronic Sensing Controls.* Philadelphia: Chilton, 1969.)

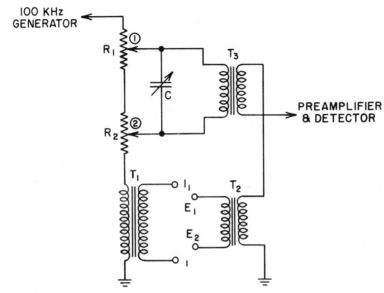

Figure 9.3 Schematic of a tetrapolar electrical impedance bridge. (Based on J. Nyboer, W. Gessert and K. A. Reid. "Counterforce ballistics in man." *Bio. Med. Sci. Instn. 4:* 42, 1968.)

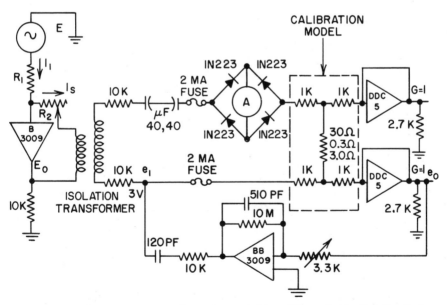

Figure 9.4 Constant current impedance bridge. (From A. Khallafalla, D. A. Spyker and S. P. Stackhouse. "Thoracic impedance techniques for the discrimination of normals from patients with chronic lung disease." *Ann. NY Acad. Sci. 170:* 689, 1970.)

PHYSIOLOGIC CALIBRATION OF TISSUE IMPEDANCE

Nyboer has developed the classic calibration experiment (Gessert, 1968). The impedance of a human leg to 100 kHz. current was measured as if it were an inorganic conductor. The resistance of a conductor = kL/A, where k = the specific resistivity of the conductor, L = the length, and A = the cross-sectional area in the direction of current flow. Connections were made to the leg by strips of aluminum foil spaced 10 cm. apart. The circumference of the leg at each foil electrode was measured for A. The constant current circuit was connected at electrodes 1 and 2, and at 3 and 4 — to each segment in turn — by connection to the adjacent aluminum strips. The bridge was balanced by successively adjusting the resistance and the capacitance until balance was attained. The resistance obtained on the calibrated resistor was plotted against calculated values of 1/A for each segment, and linear correlation was obtained.

MEASUREMENT OF RENAL BLOOD FLOW

Impedance renograms (Allison, 1966) were obtained by positioning strip electrodes across the back of the patient above and below the kidneys located by X-ray. Electrodes 3 and 4 were placed above and below the kidney, and current electrodes 1 and 2 were placed parallel to the corresponding detector electrode. When the reference signal was introduced in electrodes 1 and 2, variations in the signal obtained by electrodes 3 and 4 were attributed to changes in conductivity during each cardiac cycle. The studies were repeated for both the left and right kidney. Differences in renal blood flow were attributed to renal disease, and were confirmed by clinical examination.

Data processing included the calculation of pulse volume and flow from the ΔR obtained from each measurement. The calculated blood volume per pulse was calculated from

$$\Delta V = rL^2/\Delta R$$

where ΔV = blood volume per pulse
      r = resistivity of whole blood at 37°C (150 ohm-cm.)
      L = distance between electrodes 3 and 4

$$\Delta R = \frac{R_1 R_2}{R_1 - R_2}$$

      R_1 = resistance between electrodes 3 and 4 with no pulse (diastole)
      R_2 = resistance between electrodes 3 and 4 during systole (extrapolated)

THORACIC IMPEDANCE TECHNIQUES

We have already seen that it is difficult to obtain reproducible clinical information in diagnosing obstructive lung conditions. Impedance plethysmography has been used to provide a diagnostic tool in this area (Khallafalla, 1970). At frequencies between 60 and 280 Hz., it was found that the phase angle of impedance was less than one degree, when the resistive properties of the thorax were being monitored. Left arm, left leg, right arm, and right leg electrodes were coupled at six thoracic sites: at the second and fifth intercostal spaces, and at right, central, and left chest. The input electrodes were LA-LL or RL-RA; and across the chest they were LA-RA, LA-RL, and RA-LL.

A computer pattern recognition program was used to establish whether the tests could distinguish between normal subjects and those with chronic obstructive lung disease. The tests were performed at 280 Hz. and at 60 Hz., and an average 60 Hz. to 280 Hz. value was obtained by using a frequency adjusting factor.

It was found that the tests *could* distinguish between normal subjects and those patients with chronic obstructive lung disease, with an uncertainty of only 15%, using the computer pattern recognition program.

CARDIAC MEASUREMENTS

Impedance measurements have been made for cardiac output which agree statistically with the Fick methods or with the indicator dilution methods (Kinnen, 1970).

An impedance cardiograph has been used (Kubicek, 1970) to measure stroke volume and cardiac output according to the following formulas:

1.)
$$\Delta V = \frac{rL^2}{Z^2} T \left(\frac{dZ}{dt}\right)$$

where ΔV = stroke volume in ml.

r = resistivity of blood at 100 kHz. (150 ohm-cm.)

L = mean distance between electrodes 3 and 4 in cm.

Z = mean impedance between the electrodes 3 and 4 in ohms

$\frac{dZ}{dt}$ = minimum value of dZ/dt during cardiac cycle

T = ventricular ejection time obtained from dZ/dt curve

2.)   Cardiac Output = stroke volume × pulse rate.

Units are in ml. per minute. The detector electrodes are positioned at the base of the neck and at the lower end of the sternum; the current electrodes (1 and 2) are spaced 3 cm. beyond electrodes 3 and 4.

The dZ/dt output produces not only cardiac output and stroke volume data, but also invaluable information concerning the condition of the heart.

AUTOMATING THE CLINICAL LABORATORY

Another area benefiting from advanced applications of system theory is the clinical laboratory. We have examined various physicochemical methods of analysis, some of which can be automatically administered. We have also examined automatic applications of physicochemical analysis methods. Now, the application of time, energy, and developmental skill in automating laboratory procedures, data processing, and reporting techniques will be discussed.

AUTOMATED BLOOD ANALYSIS

The reactive photometer principle (first described by Weiss in 1954) has been used for the automated analysis of hemoglobin measurements (Fig. 9.5). Hemoglobin concentration in the blood is monitored at 548.5 mμ, at which frequency 99.5% of the hemoglobin formed in the blood absorbs electromagnetic radiation. Hemoglobin can be in its reduced form, oxidized form (oxyhemoglobin), or in combination with a toxic agent like carbon monoxide (carboxyhemoglobin).

In Figure 9.5, a pump aspirates the sample of blood through a reaction vessel with an accurately proportioned amount of hemolyzing agent. The reacted sample is passed through the cuvette in the sample area of an automatic photometer, in which a narrow band width optical

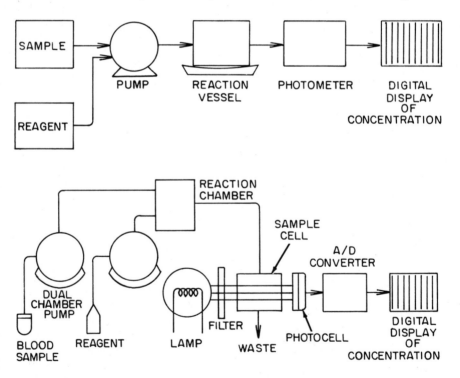

Figure 9.5 Automatic hemoglobin analysis instrumentation. *A*, Block diagram; *B*, Flow schematic.

filter provides radiation of 548.5 mμ, which is absorbed by the forms of hemoglobin in the sample. The detector photocell is connected to a digital voltmeter by circuitry calibrated to furnish direct readout in grams of hemoglobin per 100 ml. of blood.

Another routine blood analysis frequently performed is the measurement of pH, carbon dioxide, and oxygen in the blood. Instead of photometry, the electrochemical electrode technique is used; and instead of the low impedance photocell, the amplifier must be designed for a high impedance electrode. Meter display is more readily coupled with the high impedance VTVM required for electrode readout. Once the signal is amplified to the low impedance millivolt region required by the meter display, a DVM can be coupled with the system to provide digital display of pH, P_{CO_2} and P_{O_2}.

OXYGEN ELECTRODE

The Clark membrane electrode described in Chapter 5 has been improved in the 15 years since its introduction to provide more reliable and reproducible measurements of oxygen in blood. The electrode recently described (Bradley, 1966) consists of a 1 mil-platinum wire coated with glass but exposed at the tip, surrounded by a 0.1 M potassium chloride solution buffered at pH 7, and a silver/silver chloride reference electrode. The polarographic potential of -0.7 v. for oxygen is applied to the platinum cathode, and a current flow is monitored which is proportional to the oxygen concentration in the bloodstream. A polypropylene membrane covers the entire assembly to protect it from the liquids and solids in the blood. The oxygen in the blood diffuses through the membrane rapidly enough so that a satisfactory analysis is obtained.

CARBON DIOXIDE ELECTRODE

When a pH electrode is immersed in a solution of potassium chloride and sodium bicarbonate absorbed in nylon stocking material and covered with a teflon membrane, the carbon dioxide in the sample diffuses into this cell and changes its pH as a function of the P_{CO_2} in the original sample. The electrode is sensitive to carbon dioxide whether the latter is present in compressed gas, blood, liquid, or alveolar air.

pH ELECTRODE

A capillary-bore pH electrode is now commercially available with a temperature-controlled water jacket, a very small filling volume, a large sensitive area, and an open liquid junction. Reference junctions can also be obtained in a self-contained unit.

A block diagram and flow schematic of a typical blood gas analysis unit is shown in Figure 9.6.

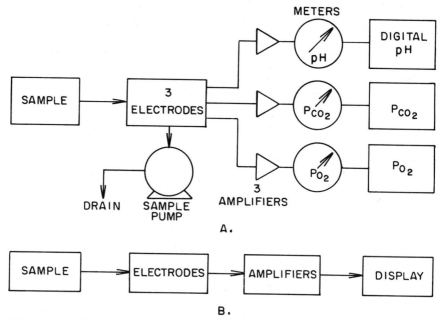

Figure 9.6 Electrochemical analysis of oxygen, carbon dioxide and pH in blood. *A*, Flow diagram; *B*, Block diagram.

DIGITAL PRINTOUT

The blood gas, or hemoglobin digital readout can now be combined with a digital computer logging system either to store the information or produce it at any location desired within the hospital. In one impressive technique, a blood sample taken from the patient before he enters the doctor's office is immediately placed into the automated instrument. While the interview proceeds, the analysis is being made, and the results are digitally coded and teletyped to the physician. He has the blood test results in hand to confirm or assist in making his clinical findings.

Less impressive results consist of a direct printout from the analyzer to accompany the patient's chart in additional interviews and procedures.

CONTINUOUS MONITORING

Continuous monitoring of P_{O_2}, P_{CO_2}, and pH using electrochemical transducers led to the development of systems for continuous monitoring of these vital parameters during and after surgery, and in intensive care units. Walton, Smith, and Wilson (1970) describe a system which is connected to the artery of the wrist to provide continuous monitoring of blood chemistry. The system is the three-electrode system already described, modified by providing for continuous blood flow through the system directly from the patient. Experience with the monitoring system showed that it helped the anesthesiologist to maintain proper pH in the patient connected to the heart-lung machine. Patients with respiratory difficulty can be monitored for the oxygen and carbon dioxide levels in their blood; the system furnishes valuable clues in maintaining the proper regimen, e.g., for endotracheal suction.

BIOMEDICAL TELEMETRY

The process of transmitting signals from a biological source to a required detector is called telemetry. The layman has become familiar with the telemetry of the physiologic parameters of the astronauts in a lunar capsule. Hence, the question is raised: "Why don't we use telemetry in the hospital and avoid all those wiring problems?"

A block diagram of a typical telemetering system is shown in Figure 9.7. In addition to the sensor, which is implanted into the patient, the primary signal must be converted to an electrical signal, amplified, modulated, amplified again, and transmitted. At the receiving end, the signal must be amplified, demodulated, amplified again, and displayed. In each area, problems arise which are unique because we are dealing with a living organism.

A simple telemetering element was used by Mackay (1959) to transmit the pressure fluctuations obtained as food moved along the gastrointestinal tract. The internal body pressure is measured by its effect on the elastic element, attached to a ferrite core which moves in the field of a coil. The rest of the circuit is an oscillator the frequency of which changes with the position of the ferrite core. The transistor provides the amplification, and the battery the power. The coil also serves

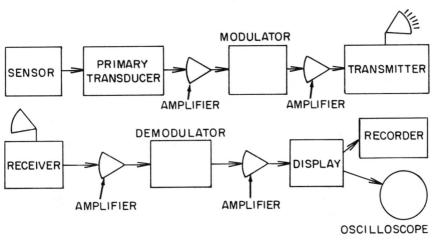

Figure 9.7 Telemetering system.

as an antenna which radiates the energy so that it can be received else-where. A Mallory 312-battery is used and will give continuous signals for about three days. Detection of the signal is by a loop antenna near the abdomen of the subject, looped over his shoulder or around his waist.

By replacing the resistor by a thermistor, and omitting the ferrite core and pressure sensor, the circuit was used to measure *temperature*.

The basic principles of transducers can be used to generate electrical signals for telemetering. Change in resistance or inductance can change a frequency, which can be transmitted to a remote point and reconverted (demodulated) to an analogue signal. These changes in carrier waves are called modulation.

MODULATION

In modulation, the character of the carrier wave is varied in accordance with the information content of another wave. The carrier wave can be modulated in one of three ways including varying its amplitude (amplitude modulation, or AM); varying its frequency (frequency modulation, or FM); or varying its phase (phase modulation, or PM).

Amplitude modulation (Fig. 9.8) is the typical radio station transmission. The sound pressure pulsations are converted to an "audio" electrical signal of 10 to 10,000 Hz., by the microphone, and this is made to modulate the amplitude of the 500 kHz. to 1000 kHz. radio signal.

Note in Figure 9.8 that all three forms of modulation are affected by the information signal.

You are probably aware that AM is "noisy," because it picks up all sorts of signals in its band. Frequency modulation is used for hi-fidelity broadcasting because it does not pick up as much noise. How-

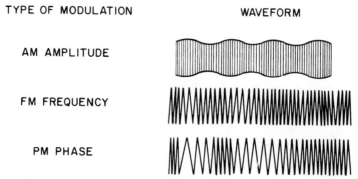

TYPE OF MODULATION   WAVEFORM

AM AMPLITUDE

FM FREQUENCY

PM PHASE

Figure 9.8 Forms of telemetry modulations. (From B. G. Lipták (ed.) *Instrument Engineers' Handbook* (Vol. II). Philadelphia: Chilton, 1970.)

ever, it is also used for television signals, in which some interference is noted from low-flying airplanes and other sources of electrical energy which in reality ought not to interfere. Briefly, this is why FM is commonly used in telemetering, where accurate signals free from noise are desired.

MULTIPLEXING

The cost of a telemetering system that sends many signals, e.g., temperature, pressure, and ECG, can be reduced considerably by using a single transmitter and receiver and multiplexing the signals. The method uses several subcarrier oscillators (SCO), each tuned to a different frequency for each variable. Their outputs are added and used to modulate the main carrier wave. After transmission and reception the mixed signal is demodulated and applied to a bank of band-pass filters tuned to the frequencies of the SCO. Each separate band-pass filter now has its own subcarrier demodulator, which provides a separate signal output. Note that both the SCO and the carrier wave are modulated and can possess either FM or AM modulation. Thus, the type of modulation is represented by a double symbol pair: the first pair representing the SCO, the second pair the carrier wave. For example, FM/AM is an AM system with FM subcarriers.

POWER SOURCES

The power source for implantable transducers has been the electro-chemical battery. Proposals have been made for utilizing atomic power, the electrochemical potential of the body, external power sources that transmit energy to the implants, the motion of the muscles to generate power, and so forth. But present telemetering devices are limited by the life of presently available batteries. A list of presently available miniature batteries furnished by Fryer (1970) in N.A.S.A. Report SP 5094 is given in Table 9.1.

SYSTEM PERFORMANCE

The basic system performance for the N.A.S.A. biopotential transmitter is given in Table 9.2 (Fryer, 1967).

The unit is roughly about the diameter of and a little thicker than a penny. The biopotentials (EEG or ECG) are preamplified and used to control an FM subcarrier oscillator, which in turn modulates a radiofrequency transmitter tuned in the 88 mega-Hz. to 108 mega-Hz. band reserved for biomedical telemetering. In the switched mode cited in Table 9.2, pulse code modulation is used instead of continuous wave. This mode of operation is useful for temperature sensing, in which a solid-state switch is controlled by a thermistor circuit. The time between the pulses is proportional to the temperature. This

TABLE 9.1 AVAILABLE BATTERIES FOR TELEMETERING SERVICE

Type	Life ma.-hr.	Maximum Current ma.	Voltage v.	Weight g.	Height cm.	Diameter cm.
RM 212	16	0.75	1.4	0.5	0.33	0.55
RM 312	36	2.0	1.4	0.56	0.34	0.77
RM 575	100	3.0	1.4	1.49	0.33	1.15
S13E	60	3.0	1.5	1.0	0.5	0.77
RM 675	160	5.0	1.4	2.2	0.54	1.16
E 301	100	0.1	1.5	1.68	0.33	1.15
E 303	165	0.24	1.5	2.5	0.5	1.15
W 1 [a]	36	0.5	1.4	0.56	0.34	0.77
W 3 [a]	165	1.0	1.4	2.24	0.5	1.15
WH 4	100	1.0	1.4	1.4	0.33	1.15
RMCC [b] 640 W	500	1.5	1.4	7.9	1.1	1.6
RMCC [b] 1W	1000	2.0	1.4	12.0	1.63	1.6

[a] These are long-life cells developed for watches.
[b] These are long-life cells developed for pacemakers.

mode of operation produces much less drain on the battery and much longer life of the transmitter.

APPLICATIONS

Since telemetry has been made available as a laboratory tool to biologists and medical researchers, hundreds of applications have been described. This section describes two of the important applications that reflect the direction and scope that this phase of biomedical instrumentation is taking.

TABLE 9.2 N.A.S.A. TRANSMITTER–SYSTEM PERFORMANCE SPECIFICATIONS

Input Impedance	20 megohms
Equivalent Input Noise	1 microvolt RMS
Frequency Response	0.5 to 120 Hz.
Power Source	1.4 volt, 36 milliampere-hour mercury cell
Battery Drain	40 microamperes pulsed, or 0.8 milliampere continuous
Size	1.9 cm. in diameter; 0.5 cm. in thickness
Weight	2 grams
System Gain	3000
Radio Frequency	88 to 108 mega-Hz.

Reproductive Biology

In reproductive biology (Balin, 1966) there is very little direct knowledge concerning follicle growth and ovulation time in the primate. To obtain some first-hand information, a temperature transmitter with the Mackay circuit was mounted next to the ovary of a rhesus monkey. Ovarian surface temperature patterns were obtained which corresponded to the different phases of the ovulatory cycle.

Behavioral Studies

Behavioral studies have been made of cats in whom stimulator electrodes have been implanted (Sperry et al., 1967). The stimulator electrode was implanted in the basomedial amygdala, which stimulates the defensive behavior of the cat. The transmitter electrode was implanted in the hypothalamus where the evoked potential from the previous stimulus is known to appear. The stimulator was a free-running multivibrator which would make the stimulator negative for 0.7 millisecond. The potentials of the hypothalamus were detected by an electrode connected to a field effect transistor (FET) which was a high impedance input to an FM transmitter.

Delgado placed a stimulating electrode in the brain of a bull and turned on the nonaggressive behavior while the bull was charging him. Fortunately, no problems developed in the telemetering system at the time.

Progress in developing a telemetry system for the intensive care area has been reported by Trummer and Reining (1969). The system transmits three channels of physiologic data and a fourth channel on the status of the battery. Body temperature, respiration rate, and ECG may be transmitted by pulse position modulation of an FM transmitter. The transmitter, which is external to the patient, is fed the data by the usual sensors: a thermistor attached to the patient's body for temperature, a nose clip thermistor for respiration, and standard ECG electrodes for brain wave activity.

PACEMAKERS

One of the medical advances which could never have happened were it not for the development of medical electronics and instrumentation is the pacemaker. The pacemaker is an implanted electronic circuit installed for the treatment of heart-block, a pathologic condition in which the A-V node ceases to function. When this happens, the ventricles are separated electrically from the atria, and beat at their own slow rate out of phase with the atrial rate. Before the introduction of the pacemaker, 50% of the patients with symptomatic heart-block died within one year.

The evolution of the pacemaker parallels that of the miniaturization of electronic instruments. At first, large external electrodes were applied to the chest, and relatively high voltage was used for stimulation (Chapter 7). The procedure was uncomfortable and painful. Internal electrodes attached directly to the heart musculature required much less voltage for stimulation. The wires from the implanted electrodes were brought through the skin to a pulse generator which was suspended by a strap against the body. To avoid the wires coming through the skin and causing infection, a radiofrequency generator was used which activated a coil under the skin. Succeeding pulse generators were made small enough to be implanted subdermally. Replacement of the battery was now a simple operation through the skin, and the disadvantages related to entry wires, or carrying an external packet were overcome.

To avoid the major operation required to implant the electrodes on the chest (thoracotomy), the through-the-vein technique was developed. The electrode was passed through the vein to the heart with the patient awake but locally anesthetized. The pulse generator was placed under the skin. This was a much less demanding procedure, especially for patients with heart-block, for whom a thoracotomy was a grave risk.

As the technique of constructing and installing pacemakers developed, the nature of the pacemaker signal itself became a significant factor. Often, as the pacemaker functioned, a normal heart rhythm returned. Now the natural beat was competing with the induced beat, and ventricular fibrillation became a potential hazard. Demand pacemakers were developed which can shut themselves off when a natural ventricular beat occurs. Standby units were developed which reduce their output signal to an ineffective level when a ventricular beat occurs. Synchronous pacemakers sense the atrial beat and stimulate a ventricular beat after an appropriate time delay. These pacemakers must be installed by opening the chest wall, since a through-the-vein method has not yet been perfected for a sensor electrode.

Temporary pacemakers may be required in myocardial infarction that leads to heart-block. A ventricular electrode is attached to an external impulse generator, and pacemaking continues until the heart-block is overcome. The external generator, and later the electrode through the vein, may be removed upon the patient's recovery. In some cases atrial pacemaking may be required, in which case the electrode is attached to the atrial epicardium.

Paired pacemaking provides an impulse soon after a paced or normal heart beat. The heart muscle is depolarized and no contraction results. It has been found, however, that the response to the next normal (or paced) impulse will have increased force. An improved heart function will have been obtained. Types of pacemakers are listed in Table 9.3.

TABLE 9.3 TYPES OF PACEMAKERS

Type	Power Supply	Rate	Electrodes	Connections
1	External	Fixed	External	
2	External	Fixed	Implanted	Wires through skin
3	Radiofrequency external	Fixed	Implanted	Inductive coils
4	Implanted under skin	Fixed	Implanted	Direct wire
5	Implanted under skin	Fixed	Venous catheter	Direct wire
6	Implanted under skin	Demand	Implanted	Direct wire
7	Implanted under skin	Standby	Implanted	Direct wire
8	Implanted under skin	Synchronous	Implanted	Wires to atrium and to ventricle

EXTERNAL ELECTRICAL STIMULATION

External electrical stimulation involves the placement of electrodes against the chest of a patient requiring emergency resuscitation for heart stoppage. About 100 volts at 50 milliamperes for 2 to 3 milliseconds has been used, providing a pulse of 0 to 400 watt-seconds of 4.7 to 5.3 milliseconds' duration. If ventricular fibrillation or other arrhythmia is present, countershock is required to stop the heart before the stimulus current can be applied. The timing of the impulse must be synchronized with the normal rhythm of the heart beat, should it resume. If not properly timed, the stimulation itself can produce ventricular fibrillation. Hence, close monitoring of the patient's ECG is required before, during, and after the external therapy is applied. The block diagram for the external stimulator then must contain the monitor as well as the stimulator (Fig. 9.9).

The external electrical pacemaker is used not only in emergencies,

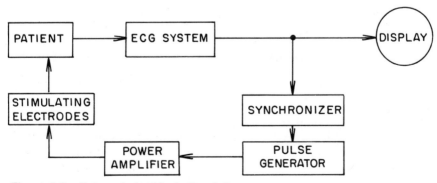

Figure 9.9 External electrical stimulation.

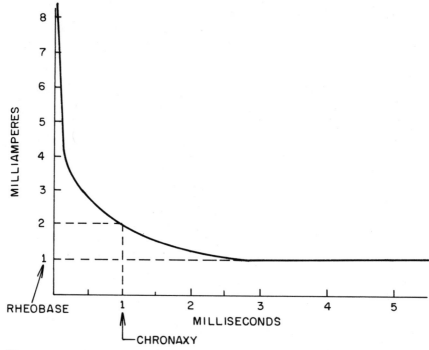

Figure 9.10 Typical strength-duration curve for a cardiac stimulus.

but also often during surgery when a pacemaker is being implanted and means are required to maintain heart function until the implant can take over.

The chronaxy is a physiologic unit of time applied to the irritability of cells. For the heart musculature it reflects the strength–duration relationship of signals which would produce response. The minimum stimulus must be present at the heart muscle to produce desired response. A typical strength–duration curve is shown in Figure 9.10. The minimum current has an asymptote at long duration called the rheobase. The chronaxy is defined as the time at which a stimulus just double the rheobase has to be applied to evoke a response. Thus, in Figure 9.10, the rheobase is 1 milliampere. The chronaxy would be a stimulus of 2 milliamperes which must be sustained for 1 millisecond to produce a response.

DIRECT WIRE STIMULATION

In postsurgical heart-block, the electrode can be inserted into the heart by a needle proceeding from the skin (percutaneous) through the chest to the heart. The heart electrical impulse indicates passage through the wall (pericardium) into the muscle (myocardium). When the tip of the needle has penetrated the heart muscle, a fine stainless steel wire is slipped through the needle and left in the heart when the needle is withdrawn. External pacemaking is provided until the patient recovers, following which the electrode can be removed (ref. Lillehei).

TRANSVENOUS CONNECTION

An alternate procedure to direct wire stimulation is to introduce a catheter electrode into the right ventricle by way of the jugular vein by the standard heart catheterization procedure. The tip is located by fluoroscopic monitoring, and electrical monitoring is done at the same time to see whether the proper heart impulse is being received. Braided wire core with platinum contacts seems to offer the best results. A standard pacemaker is attached and suspended from the patient's neck. The catheter may have only one pole, with a return circuit to the skin, or it may be bipolar. Maintenance currents of 2 to 4 ma. are often used. A silver ground plate against the skin spreads the area of contact so that the sticking feeling from the current is removed (Escher).

RADIOFREQUENCY INDUCTIVE STIMULATION

When heart-block is present and long-term pacemaking is required, a radiofrequency stimulator with implanted electrodes in the right ventricle provides ready battery replacement. The electrodes are implanted by a thoracotomy, and the leads are brought out through the skin for cardiac stimulation during the early postoperative period. A radio receiver is implanted under the skin and connected to the left heart by separate electrodes. The antenna from the radiowave transmitter is taped to the skin over the site of the receiver, and the transmitter is held in a pocket in an undervest. The radiofrequency (R-F) signal is transmitted not continuously, but for one millisecond out of each second. The pulse rate may be adjusted by changing the timing of the master switch which activates the R-F transmission of a two-megacycle signal (ref. Widmann).

An alternate R-F pacemaker of Italian design (Cammilli) has a receiver coil implanted on the heart. Rectangular pulses 1 to 10 milliseconds in width are transmitted with a rhythm variable from 30 to 150 impulses per minute. The R-F transmission is in the 4 to 5 mega-Hz. region. The position of the coil on the heart is selected so that a short direct R-F transmission route with the external pacemaker is available.

IMPLANTABLE PACEMAKERS

The next step in the history of pacemakers was to develop a pacemaker circuit which would be sufficiently reliable to implant inside the body, and draw very little current so that it would provide long battery life. A circuit like that shown in Figure 9.11 was used, designed so that it could be triggered by magnetic induction through the abdominal wall to vary the heart rate from 64 to 120 pulses per minute.

The electrodes are implanted in the left ventricle, and wires run to the unit placed under the skin. The external control unit is taped to the outside of the skin opposite the internal unit (Kantrowitz). An alternate approach (Zoll) uses no external elements and a fixed rate of 70 pulses per minute (15 ma., 2 msec.).

The synchronous pacemaker (Nathan) requires an atrial electrode which picks up the 2.5 mv. atrial P-wave and two ventricular electrodes. The pacemaker is placed in the abdomen, below the belt, and wires lead from the heart electrodes to the implanted pacemaker. The block diagram of the pacemaking system is shown in Figure 9.11. Elements include a P-wave amplifier, an A-V delay, a logic block, and an output amplifier. The logic block provides an output in response to the atrial signal unless atrial fibrillation is occurring, in which case a fixed signal of 52 pulses per minute is sent to the ventricles. Atrial rates slower than 52, or P-waves below the sensing capabilities of the

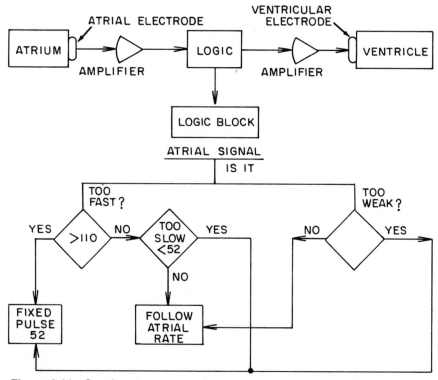

Figure 9.11 Synchronous pacemaker system.

amplifier, will result in synchronous pulses being emitted by the logic block. Thus, forms of failure other than A-V heart-block will be compensated for by this pacer unit.

ENGINEERING PROBLEMS IN PACEMAKER FABRICATION

Engineering problems in pacemaker fabrication, in addition to the medical problems already discussed, include electrode failure due to fatigue as the heart beats regularly and rapidly and bends the electrode at each beat; and leakage of the pacemaker case, which commonly results in the body fluids' attacking the internal circuitry of the pacemaker and damaging it.

The electrode problem seems to be solved by the use of platinum electrodes, implanted in such a way that a minimum of stress is applied with each heart beat. The encapsulation problem is solved by the use of an epoxy inner case for support and complete sealing, surrounded by a silastic outer case that is compatible with body tissues.

SUMMARY

The application of impedance bridges to the measurement of changes in the volume of parts of the body constitutes impedance plethysmography. The developers of this analytical tool have measured the changes in the impedance of tissues with a pulse of blood flow through those tissues. They have measured the flow of blood through the kidneys, and the output, stroke volume, and condition of the heart.

System analysis has applied instrumental techniques to the clinical laboratory. The reactive photometer principle has been applied to hemoglobin measurements. Electrochemical techniques make use of oxygen, carbon dioxide, and pH electrodes in blood gas analysis. Digital printout provides a numerical result for the physician's records. Continuous monitoring of patients with respiratory difficulties can underline the need for endotracheal suction or other clinical management.

Biomedical telemetry has become miniaturized as microelectronics has developed. Miniature electrodes are now available for the transmission of signals based on the transducer sensors described in earlier chapters, pressure–temperature relationships, flow, and biopotentials.

The pacemaker has become the mechanism of choice for the reversal of heart-block, i.e., when the A-V node refuses to transmit its electrical signal. Internal electrodes directly attached to the heart musculature reduce the need for high currents. Small pulse generators can be implanted under the skin, and batteries readily replaced by a simple operation. Pervenous electrodes are inserted through the veins to avoid an extensive thoracotomy. Fixed pacing has been supplemented by demand pacing for hearts that occasionally resume their pumping action.

EXERCISES

1. Consult section on renal blood flow to calculate the resistance change for normal renal blood flow if the impedance plethysmography electrodes are spaced 1 inch apart.

2. Using standard stroke volume of the heart, apply the equation given to calculate the impedance (dZ/dt) measured by the impedance cardiograph with L at distance of 1 inch. (Hint: assume Z = 100 ohms.)

3. A standard sample of blood containing 15 g. of hemoglobin per 100 ml. blood registered 152 mv. on the automatic photometer. If the digital voltmeter (DVM) has an infinite input impedance, what gain should be placed on the A/D converter to provide direct reading on the 0 to 100 volt DVM?

4. The oxygen electrode in the same blood standard from question 3 registers 600 mv. If the oxygen saturation is 100% of this sample, what mv. signal would the electrode read at 50% saturation? (Hint: electrode potential follows Nernst's equation.)

5. The pH reading is 7.36. What can you tell about the blood sample? Is it arterial or venous blood? Is its pH normal, high, or low?

6. It is desired to monitor the pH of the blood of a polar bear before, during, and after hibernation. Design a telemetering system for the experiment, using the principles outlined in this chapter.

7. It is desired to determine where salmon go when they swim out to sea after emerging from their river habitat. There are many places along the river where the salmon can be trapped, and telemetering devices inserted under the integument. Comment on the odds of following a signal by means of directional antenna on shore and aboard ship from a school of salmon during their ocean migration. What type of telemetering device would tend to be most successful in this regard?

8. Select the proper battery from Table 9.1 for each of the following applications: a.) A pacemaker, which draws 0.1 ma. of current for each heart beat; b.) An astronaut's ECG transmitter required to send a continuous signal for a twelve-hour orbit around the earth. The apparatus requires 14 v. to operate, and no more than 2 lbs. is allowable for batteries. The instrument requires 0.1 ma. of current for each P-QRS-T complex transmitted.

9. Something has gone wrong with the logic circuit of the synchronous pacer system in Figure 9.11 in that there are two pulses stimulating the ventricle—the fixed pulse and the synchronous pulse. What do you think has gone wrong and how would you correct it?

General Literature Cited and References

Albert, H. M., Glass, B. A., Pittman, B., and Robichaux, P. Cardiac stimulation threshold: acute studies. *Ann. NY Acad. Sci. 111*:889, 1964.

Allison, R. D. (editor) Bioelectric Impedance Measurements of Cardiac Output, Lung Volumes and the Cerebral Circulation. Pittsburgh: ISA, 1970.

Allison, R. D. Recent biomedical applications of four-electrode impedance measuring techniques. *Bio. Med. Sci. Instn. 3*:309, 1966.

Ballin, H. Telemetry and reproductive biology. *Bio. Med. Sci. Instn. 3*:113, 1966.

Caceres, C. (editor) Biomedical Telemetry. New York: Academic, 1965.

Cammilli, L., Pozzi, R., Pissichi, G., and De Saint-Pierre, G. Radiofrequency pacemaker with receiver coil implanted in the heart. Ann. NY Acad. Sci. 111:1007, 1964.

Chardack, W. M. A myocardial electrode for long-term pacemaking. Ann. NY Acad. Sci. 111:893, 1964.

Delgado, J. M. R. Stimulating and Recording Electrodes. In Physical Techniques in Biological Research. New York: Academic, 1964.

Escher, D. Transvenous electrical stimulation of the heart. Ann. NY Acad. Sci. 111:972, 1964.

Fryer, T. B. Implantable Biotelemetry Systems. Washington: NASA, 1970.

Fryer, T. B. Survey of biomedical instrumentation development at Ames research center. Bio. Med. Sci. Instn. 3:113, 1966.

Geddes, L. A. The Measurement of Physiological Events by Impedance. In F. Alt (editor) Advances in Bioengineering and Instrumentation. New York: Plenum, 1966.

Gessert, W. L., Reid, K. A., and Nyboer, J. Reliability of tetrapolar electrical impedance plethysmography. Bio. Med. Sci. Instn. 5:143, 1964.

Glenn, W. W. L. (editor) Cardiac Pacemakers. New York: NY Academy of Science, 1964.

Kastor, J. J., and Harthorne, J. W. Types of cardiac pacing. Proceedings of the 8th International Conference on Medical and Biological Engineering: 29-1, 1969.

Khallafalla, A., Spyker, D. A., and Stackhouse, S. P. Thoracic impedance techniques for the discrimination of normals from patients with chronic lung disease. Ann. NY Acad. Sci. 170:689, 1970.

Kinnen, E. Impedance measurements of cardiac output. In R. D. Allison (editor). Bioelectric Impedance Measurements of Cardiac Output, Lung Volumes and the Cerebral Circulation. Pittsburgh: ISA, 1970.

Lillehei, C. W. Control of complete heart block by means of an artificial pacemaker and myocardial electrodes. Circ. Res. 6:410, 1958.

Mackay, R. S. Biomedical Telemetry. New York: Wiley, 1970.

Myers, G. H., and Parsonnet, V. Cardiac pacemakers. In Y. Nose, Cardiac Engineering. New York: Interscience, 1970.

Nathan, D. A., et al. Application of a cardiac synchronous pacer for the correction of Stokes-Adams attacks. Ann. NY Acad. Sci. 111:1093, 1964.

Nyboer, J. Electrical Impedance Plethysmography. Springfield, Ill.: Thomas, 1959.

Slater, L. (editor) Biotelemetry. New York: Pergamon, 1963.

Sperry, C. J., et al. Implantable stimulator and transmitter for telemetry of evoked potentials during defensive behavior. Bio. Med. Sci. Instn. 4:119, 1967.

Trummer, J. R., and Reining, W. N. A four channel telemetry system for intensive care. Proceedings of the 8th International Conference on Medical and Biological Engineering: 30-6, 1969.

Whelan, R. E., et al. Electrical hazards associated with cardiac pacemaking. Ann. NY Acad. Sci. 111:922, 1964.

Widmann, W. D., et al. Radiofrequency cardiac pacemakers. Ann. NY Acad. Sci. 111:992, 1964.

Zoll, P. M. Implantable cardiac pacemakers. Ann. NY Acad. Sci. 111:1068, 1964.

Zoll, P. M. Resuscitation of heart in ventricular standstill by external electrode stimulation. New Eng. J. Med. 247:768, 1952.

Chapter 10

Biomedical Systems Development

WE NOW HAVE the tools to build biomedical instrumentation systems. They include electronics, transducers, the principles of physiology, an understanding of medical problems, electrochemical transducers, electromagnetic absorption and other physicochemical techniques, the bedside monitors that record the vital signs, diagnostic instruments that warn us of the advent of pathologic states, subsystems for automating the analysis, telemetering signals from inside the body, and pacemakers for maintaining the heart in its rhythmic state despite damage to its conduction mechanism.

But do we have all the tools we need? We are missing the cement that ties together the complex system that satisfies a requirement. This binding material is the technology of systems engineering, and the analog and digital computer that will supply the calculation and control required for the system to operate.

PRINCIPLES OF SYSTEMS ENGINEERING

Systems engineering received its initial impetus during World War II with the construction of electronic devices (radar, sonar, loran) for the military. It was utilized in the extensive development and design of the atomic bomb; the lunar space program; the digital computer; chemical, industrial, and operational processes; and now, biomedical systems.

The procedure has been standardized, and by means of block diagrams, programmed evaluation review techniques (PERT), and critical path methods (CPM), the course of a project can be estimated and its progress revised. A checklist of priorities should be prepared and followed so that the project can proceed smoothly.

Systems engineering can be illustrated by a series of block diagrams demonstrating both the overall view and the steps that comprise it.

Figure 10.1 shows the phases, steps, parts, and tools. Each phase of systems engineering has an exterior part and an interior part. The

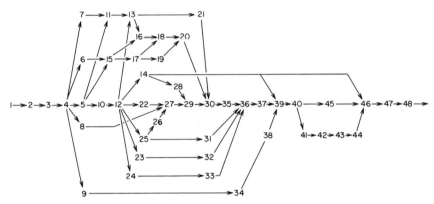

1 Evaluate feasibility	24 Specify and order new sensors
2 Write and send out specification	25 Specify cables and other wiring
3 Evaluate bids and select vendor	26 Manufacture cables
4 Form project team	27 Assemble hardware
5 Review system functions	28 Build or procure test equipment
6 Take system design course	29 Check equipment in vendor's shop
7 Take programing course	30 Check system in vendor's shop
8 Take maintenance course	31 Do on-site wiring
9 Start management and operator familiarization	32 Prepare site and modify plant
10 Review equipment requirements	33 Install new sensors
11 Make general plans for programming	34 Prepare operator manuals
12 Specify input-output terminal locations	35 Ship hardware
13 Assign input-output memory locations	36 Connect hardware at site
14 Specify factory and field test procedures	37 Check noncontrol functions
15 Develop first control function(s)	38 Train operators
16 Program first control function(s)	39 Perform equipment acceptance tests
17 Develop second control function(s)	40 Check first control function(s)
18 Program second control function(s)	41 Collect data
19 Develop third control function(s)	42 Develop new control functions
20 Program third control function(s)	43 Program new control functions
21 Program executive and noncontrol functions	44 Check new control functions
22 Manufacture or procure special equipment	45 Check other control functions
23 Specify site details and plant modifications	46 Perform functional acceptance test
	47 Evaluate system performance
	48 Improve and expand system

Figure 10.1 An overall look at systems engineering. (From B. G. Lipták (ed.) *Instrument Engineers' Handbook* (Vol. II). Philadelphia: Chilton, 1970.)

exterior part involves concepts outside the solution to the project, e.g., the statement of the problem and procedures for solving it. The interior part involves the actual solutions to the problem.

PHASES OF SYSTEM DESIGN

The phases of system design illustrate the chronological order in which a project should be carried out, and the stepwise development by which a solution is sought. When experienced engineers are first exposed to this procedure they often comment, "But isn't this what we have always done?" If they are successful engineers, undoubtedly this is the procedure they have followed, for it is a logical, efficient way to complete a job. Just as the surgeon establishes a procedure for each type of surgical treatment, so the systems engineer develops a procedure for each project, and the procedures all contain the same six phases.

Phase I. Initiation

To start the project the engineer requires a clear statement of the problem and a specific list of possible solutions. In addition to defining the problem, a measure to gauge the effectiveness of the solution is needed. The initial phase often starts with a person who suddenly sees a problem clearly and at the same time thinks that he sees a way to solve it. He talks to anyone he can find with expert opinion on the subject, consults the bibliography, attends meetings at which discussion of solutions to other problems may help him with his, marshals all his resources to obtain a solution without divulging the problem needlessly. When he feels that he has sufficiently explored various avenues of approach and has an inkling to a solution, he writes an initiation report in the form of a proposal. It contains 1.) a clear statement of the problem, and 2.) a test method that it is felt will provide a solution. These are the external parts of the proposal. The internal parts are concerned with the manner of solving the problem. What are the possible approaches to a solution? Which of them are the more effective? What is the probability of success of each? What is the estimated cost? What are the estimated returns? The returns may not be monetary, at least not directly. That is, there may be manpower savings, or reduction in nurses' or laboratory time. Lives may be saved.

The product of the initiation phase is a report. If the report is convincing, administrative channels will probably approve the report and allow continuance of the project. If the report is not convincing, the project stops at this point.

Phase II. Organization

If approval is obtained, the project leader proceeds to organize the team necessary for implementing the project. He lists the experts and specialists required for each phase of the project, the approximate date by which they will be needed, and the duration for which they will be required. He proposes a plan for the execution of the project in the form of block diagrams, PERT, and CPM charts. He reviews the three steps in exterior design (statement of the problem, formulation of mathematical models, and design of test experiments). He then considers the three steps in interior design (the single thread, high traffic, and competitive stages).

In exterior design he will require a statement of the overall problem and statements of subsidiary problems that may be encountered. He outlines the nature of the overall mathematical model and lists the mathematical models of the parts of the problem that must be developed. He describes the type of experiments that will have to be performed in order to evaluate each mathematical model, and the experiments that will be performed later to evaluate each device that has to be built.

For the interior design he needs to outline the three steps to be undertaken. Will he have single thread design, high traffic design, or competitive design? Single thread design is the design of a single unit which must function by itself. High traffic design involves concepts like queuing theory, i.e., will the system be able to cope with the traffic load imposed on it? For example, not only must we design a bedside monitor, but we must design a central station that will handle the traffic of information coming from the bedside monitors. The third step is competitive design. In industry this means competition with other companies, domestic and foreign, in the same field. In military systems this means competition with the enemy; but in medical systems this may mean competition with Death. Will the system be operable in time to save the patient's life? Will information from a complex system of many patients be sufficient to afford each patient timely protection? Game theory is invaluable in providing a mathematical tool that can help answer such questions.

The product from Phase II is another report. It will contain a list of personnel and equipment required, a plan for acquisition of materials, a time schedule for men and materials, and a list of solutions to be undertaken, with their priorities and the procedure for undertaking each. Which is the preferred path and how should it be started? The time schedule will include curves for required money, personnel, and materials. If the report is approved, the team leader proceeds to collect his team and begins the project.

Phase III. Preliminary Design

The preliminary design phase means "do the job." But because the problems and the solutions are difficult, and the end result not always attainable, the word "preliminary" is usually required. The various studies for the first, second, and third alternate designs are undertaken, and from their conclusions a preliminary design for a system that will produce the desired result is obtained. Often during this phase, changes are made in the ultimate goal, including the definition of the project, its measure of effectiveness, or the selection of the approach to follow.

All those with expertise draw on their individual specialties to produce a simulated solution. Very often the simulated solution is tried on a computer or in the form of another model.

In phase three the team goes through the exterior aspects, the interior aspects, and the subsystem parts of the project.

The product of Phase III is still another report. This time the report is a comprehensive list of specifications for the construction of a model of the system. If the design and specifications are approved, the project leader takes the project from the designers and moves it into the construction and test phase. His report will contain a proposal for the next step including what needs to be constructed, and how soon; what men, materials, and test facilities will be needed; how long construction will take; and how this plan correlates with the original plan.

Phase IV. Preliminary Test

In the model shop, preliminary prototypes of the final design are built. These are installed in a captive hospital or clinic, and the prototype is evaluated. Field experiments are designed and evaluated by computers, and the various subsystems are constructed, tested, and rated. The product of this phase is a report on the effectiveness of the product and a proposal for additional action. Should the project be abandoned? Should it be changed? Should it be carried out as originally planned? The report and its recommendations are forwarded to the proper personnel and approval is received to continue with the final design.

Phase V. Principal Design

The design team is again reassembled, modified on the basis of the previous tests. Exterior, interior, and subsystem parts are designed and built, and a final prototype prepared. This phase requires more time than any of the others, but its description is very brief. A report is prepared that contains all the plans and specifications for purchase and construction of the final unit. It is forwarded through the necessary channels and, if approved, proceeds to the purchasing and manufacturing department for implementation.

Phase VI. Construction and Test

The final unit is constructed and subjected to the tests proposed, e.g., the satellite is placed in orbit or sent to the moon; the automated multiphasic patient examination facility is built and tested; the new telemetry system is installed in a hospital and used for monitoring the critically ill patients; or a new pacemaker is implanted and works successfully in animals.

Whatever the project, the final test is the important phase. If it is successful, there may not be another report, merely a product or system that is now operative. Usually, there is a final report that indicates what went wrong, what did not work, and what must be done in the next project. Quite frequently, another initiation report is written which proposes another approach or idea which appeared during this phase of the project.

COMPUTER SYSTEMS

Computer systems may be divided into analog computer systems and digital computer systems. Analog computer systems deal with a signal which continuously changes to indicate a variable in the process. Digital computer systems represent the variables in a process by numbers, which can be recognized and modified by the computer. Numbers may be the ordinary decimal variety, expressed in engineering units; more commonly they are binary numbers. The electronic components of the digital computer, having only two states, can deal effectively with the 0 or 1 of the binary number system. The analog system is a network of components attached to operational amplifiers and can handle continuous variation in voltages, the voltages being the analog or machine representation of the process variable.

Analog computers are used to solve differential equations. Digital computers are used to solve numerical equations. Analog computers are used to develop and represent dynamic models of systems, whereas digital computers are used to process data, do numerical calculations, and carry out logical operations.

ANALOG COMPUTERS

The basic building block of the analog computer is the operational amplifier, which differs from the amplifier attached to record players and electric guitars in that it must handle DC signals. The signals used in the analog computer are slowly varying DC signals of 100 Hz. or lower. The operational amplifier must have high DC gain (e.g., 600 million), low drift (e.g., less than 1 mv. per second), and low noise (less than 15 mv. in a 100 v. signal). To obtain such characteristics, operational amplifiers use regulated power supplies, differential input stages, and stable high-precision resistors and capacitors. Most units employ automatic stabilization circuits, and some use chopper stabilizers. A typical DC operational amplifier with chopper stabilization is shown in Figure 10.2, and the symbol for the circuit is shown in Figure 10.3. An input impedance network of resistors and

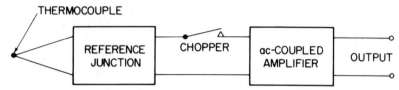

Figure 10.2 Operational amplifier with chopper stabilization. (From S. E. Summer *Electronic Sensing Controls*. Philadelphia: Chilton, 1969.)

capacitors is represented by Z_i, and a feedback impedance of resistors and capacitors is represented by Z_f.

By using various arrangements of resistors and capacitors in the input and feedback impedances, the operational amplifier can be used as a sign inverter, summer, integrator, or summing integrator. In preparing logic diagrams of computer operations, the shorthand symbols shown in Figure 10.5 are useful.

POTENTIOMETERS

The potentiometer is a component of analog computation. The term has also been used to represent "potential metering," and it has the same function on the analog computer. It is an accurately wound rheostat, in which the slide wire is activated to a specific potential, a portion of which is tapped off by the moveable slider. The potentiometer is used to multiply a variable by a constant less than 1. If the variable at a given point is 10 v., and the potentiometer is set at 0.5 of range, the output would be 5 v. We have multiplied the variable by a constant a less than 1. The circuit and the symbol for a potentiometer are shown in Figure 10.6.

To multiply two variables together, the potentiometer would not work unless we used a servomotor to move the slider on it. Such a device is called a servopotentiometer, and its mode of operation and symbol are shown in Figure 10.7. The servopotentiometer has been replaced in more modern units with quarter-square multipliers. By using the arrangement shown in Figure 10.8, one can continuously multiply two variables without moving any sliding contacts. This

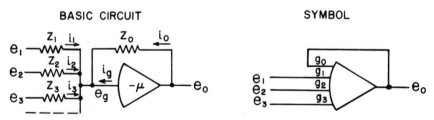

Figure 10.3 Operational amplifier. (From B. G. Lipták (ed.) *Instrument Engineers' Handbook* (Vol. II). Philadelphia: Chilton, 1970.)

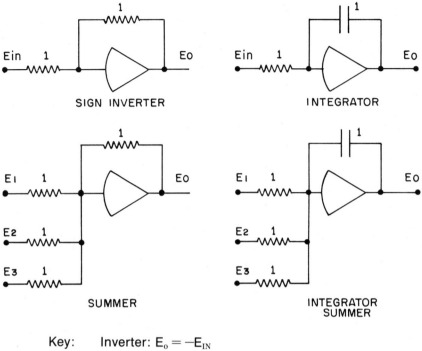

Key: Inverter: $E_o = -E_{IN}$
        Summer: $E_o = -(E_1 + E_2 + E_3)$
        Integrator: $E_o = -\int E_{IN}dt$
        Integrator Summer: $E_o = -\int (E_1 + E_2 + E_3)dt$

Figure 10.4 Impedance arrangement of operational amplifier for various computational tasks.

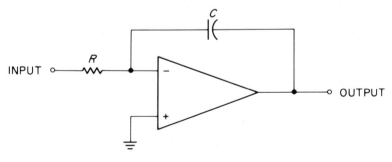

Figure 10.5 Shorthand symbols for various operational amplifier uses. (From S. E. Summer *Electronic Sensing Controls*. Philadelphia: Chilton, 1969.)

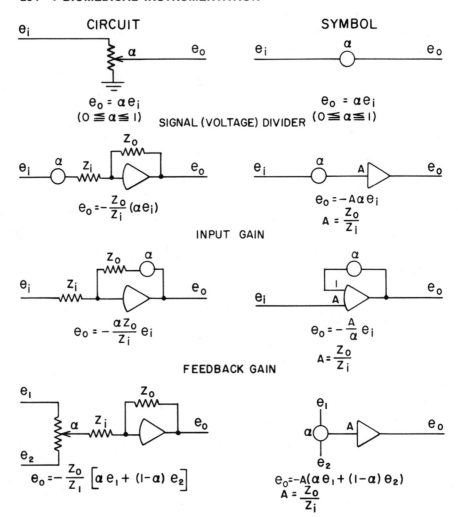

Figure 10.6 Operation and symbols for a potentiometer. (From B. G. Lipták (ed.) *Instrument Engineers' Handbook* (Vol. II). Philadelphia: Chilton, 1970.)

leads to a more reliable computational system. The quarter-square multiplier is based on the identity:

$$XY = \frac{(X + Y)^2 - (X - Y)^2}{4}$$

because if the squares are multiplied,

$$(X + Y)^2 = X^2 + 2XY + Y^2$$

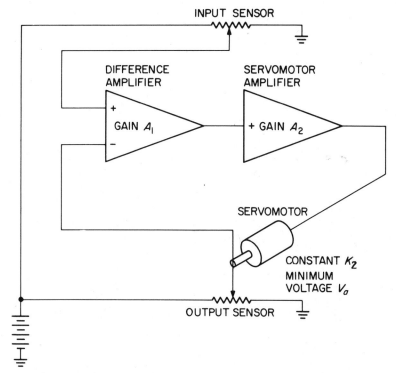

Figure 10.7 Operation and symbols for a servopotentiometer. (From S. E. Summer *Electronic Sensing Controls.* Philadelphia: Chilton, 1969.)

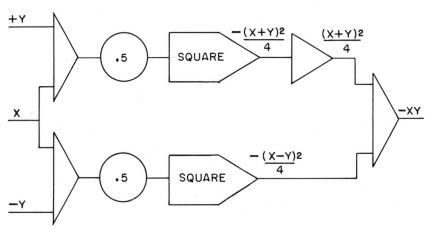

Figure 10.8 Quarter-square multiplier.

and

$$(X - Y)^2 = X^2 - 2XY + Y^2$$

And if the second expression is subtracted from the first, 4XY is obtained.

NONLINEAR FUNCTIONS

The quarter-square multiplier is operable because it is possible to build a solid-state squarer whose output is the square of its input. It uses the principle of a nonlinear function generator (NLFG). The NLFG produces a variable Y which is any function of X that can be plotted in curve form. The NLFG has a series of diodes which serve to approximate the curve by a series of straight lines. With enough line segments, the curve can be matched accurately. In the squarer, the output is the square of the input as approximated by a series of straight lines. The symbols for nonlinear operation are shown in Figure 10.9, with specific symbols for the individual NLFG's normally supplied with an analog computer.

The main application of the analog computer is in the solution of differential equations. The differential equation is manipulated so that

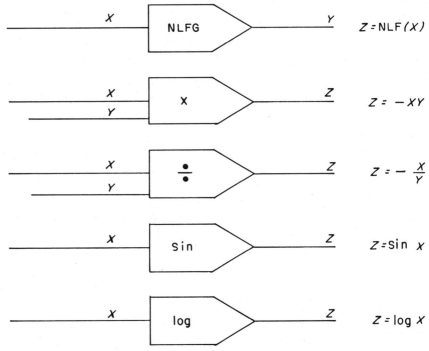

Figure 10.9 Symbols for nonlinear functions.

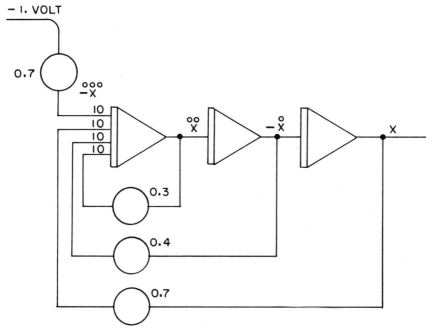

Figure 10.10 Analog computer diagram of a third-order equation.

everything but the largest derivative is on the right-hand side. The equation then reflects the patching of the input to that derivative. A simple example will demonstrate the point.

Given the equation:

$$\frac{d^3x}{dt^3} + 3\frac{d^2x}{dt^2} + 4\frac{dx}{dt} + 7x = 7$$

the transformation for programming is

$$-\frac{d^3x}{dt^3} = 3\frac{d^2x}{dt^2} + 4\frac{dx}{dt} + 7x - 7$$

We assume that all the derivatives exist and can be obtained by the use of integrations by the analog computer. That is, the $\frac{d^2x}{dt^2} = \int \frac{d^3x}{dt^3}$, and so on. Figure 10.10 represents the analog computer diagram of the equation. Note that each amplifier produces an inversion in sign. From Figure 10.10 it can be seen that in order to obtain a multiplier greater than 1.0, we use a potentiometric setting of $1/10$ and an amplifier gain of 10, obtained by making $Z_f/Z_i = 10$. The constant value 7 is obtained by a potentiometer set at 0.7 and a gain of 10 on the amplifier.

CARDIOVASCULAR CIRCULATION SIMULATION

To show how this system can be used to study cardiovascular circulation, we recall that flow $= \dfrac{\text{driving force}}{\text{resistance}}$, and that driving force = blood pressure differential.

In outline form, the blood in cardiovascular circulation is routed, starting with the left heart, as follows: from the left heart (L) to the systemic arteries (SA) to the systemic veins (SV) to the right heart (R) to the pulmonary trunk (P) and back again to the left heart. Flow equations derived from this circulation include

1.) $$\frac{dV_{SA}}{dt} = F_L - \frac{P_A - P_V}{R}$$

The change in volume of blood in the arteries = flow in − flow out. Change in volume in the veins = flow in − flow out.

2.) $$\frac{dV_V}{dt} = \frac{P_A - P_V}{R_S} - F_R$$

3.) $$\frac{dV_R}{dt} = F_{R_{in}} - F_{R_{out}} \quad \text{change in volume of right heart}$$

4.) $$\frac{dV_P}{dt} = F_{R_{out}} - \frac{P_{PA} - P_{PV}}{R_P} \quad \begin{array}{l}\text{change in volume of}\\ \text{pulmonary system}\end{array}$$

5.) $$\frac{dV_{PV}}{dt} = \frac{P_{PA} - P_{PV}}{R_p} - F_{L_{in}}$$

6.) $$\frac{dV_L}{dt} = F_{L_{in}} - F_{L_{out}}$$

The flows are sometimes zero, e.g.,

F_{in} to right or left heart = zero during systole; otherwise = $P_{sv} - P_r$ or $P_{pv} - P_L$

F_{out} of right or left heart = zero during diastole $= \dfrac{\pi}{2T_s} SV \sin \dfrac{\pi}{T_s} t$

if the duration of systole be T_s and of the entire heart cycle $T = \dfrac{60}{HR}$

HR = heart rate in beats per minute; SV = stroke volume

The stroke volumes, by Starling's law, are proportional to the heart volumes, $SV = S(V - V_0)$. The pressure in each heart and circulatory chamber is related to the volume by the compliance of that chamber (as long as the volume is stretched beyond the relaxation capacity V_0 of that chamber).

$$P_{SA} = \frac{V_{SA} - V_o}{C_{SA}} + (P_o)_{SA}$$

$$(P - P_o)_{SV} = \frac{(V - V_o)_{SV}}{C_{SV}} \qquad \text{same equation for right heart, left heart,}$$

pulmonary veins, and pulmonary arteries.

The six different blood volumes represent six variables, six integrations which can be programmed to represent the entire circulatory system.

Studies of the circulatory system have been made on such a simulation by McLaughlin (1970) to demonstrate the recovery of the circulatory system from real or imagined conditions, such as pooling of blood in the veins or arteries, or recovery from a sudden hemorrhage. The ability of the reflexes to restore arterial pressure and the effect of heart rate on mean arterial pressure, stroke volume, and cardiac output can all be investigated by means of this model.

THE DIGITAL COMPUTER

The digital computer is a high-speed electronic calculator, which has a memory bank in which the commands for the computer can be stored. It has logic which can select commands from several paths. It has output capability of typing or printing data at a very rapid speed. The most useful functions of the digital computer are monitoring, computation, control, and simulation.

MONITORING

The digital computer can be connected to a source of data, collect and store the data, and act on alarm sources in the data according to any logic conceived by the programmer. Thus, the digital computer can collect ECG's from all over the country, analyze them according to a specified procedure, store the results with the identification of the patient, and send the results of the analysis by teletype or telephone anywhere in the country.

The digital computer can, for example, collect data about hours of work, weekly rates, and so on, store the information until needed, and when needed, rapidly calculate the payroll for a large organization.

COMPUTATION

The digital computer, according to its second function, is a computer. It can add rapidly. All other functions of the computer are performed by multiple addition (multiplication), addition of complements (subtraction), or multiple addition of complements (division). The computer calculates logarithms or trigonometric functions either by some approximate calculation or by "table look up." In the latter procedure, the information is readily available in tabular form within the machine.

DIGITAL CONTROL

The digital computer can control by following orders, without demur or error. To control the temperature of a furnace, for instance, the digital computer has an input signal, resulting from the analog-to-digital conversion of the temperature sensed by a thermocouple. It compares that input signal to another number, the desired temperature, which may be calculated from the outside air temperature, the relative humidity in the building, the season of the year, and the time of day. It can then move the controls of the furnace in accordance with an algorithm (algebraic equation) which has been fed to it. It can increase or decrease the temperature at a specific rate, proportional to the deviation, the integral of the deviation, the rate of the deviation, or a combination of all three.

SIMULATION

Simulation on the digital computer involves replacing a physical event by its mathematical equivalent, and performing an analysis on that equivalent. A complete industrial machine shop can be represented by a series of storage cells in the computer's memory. Products can be fabricated in the plant in accordance with an annual schedule. Tabs can be kept on the waiting time of each machine and the waiting line before each machine. A one-year estimate can be made of the efficiency with which the machine shop can process the particular product mix. The same simulation (called a Monte Carlo simulation) can be performed with other arrangements of machines and other product mixes to determine the optimum combination for that shop.

HOW IT WORKS

How does a digital computer perform all these tasks? It has hardware and software. The hardware comprises the circuits, wires, printers, wheels, and lights that perform the task, and can be subdivided into input, arithmetic/logic, control, storage, and output. The input/output functions may be performed by a single element in the computer system—a card punch/reader, for example, a typewriter console, or a magnetic tape unit.

The card punch/reader is a unit that can read cards to communicate with the machine (input); or it can punch cards to reflect what the machine has calculated (output). The program is card-punched in code (e.g., Fortran). When punched in Fortran, each card is an equation, a command, or a reference statement. The reader converts the holes in the cards to a machine language (binary) code, and stores the information in the computer's memory. After the last Fortran card has been stored (and checked for errors by the machine), an end statement is made which tells the machine to compile.

The computer translates each card statement into many machine language statements. When it completes the compilation, it reads the data required and performs the calculations according to the program it has just compiled. As it performs the calculations, it produces the data required by 1.) punching an output card; 2.) recording the data by high-speed printer; or 3.) reproducing it on a typewriter. If it is a very high-speed machine it will place the data on a magnetic tape for subsequent playback by a slower machine.

The control unit of the machine closes the proper switches to carry out the necessary operations. For example, upon reading a program, it will close the switch to place the information from the cards into the proper sequence of spaces in memory. Upon compiling a program, it will find the compiler program on the large-scale storage unit (the disk), and place it in memory (the high-speed random access core unit). Having done so, it will return to the first compiler instruction and carry it out. The instruction may say, "read the first statement of the Fortran program," and based on what that statement is take certain actions. Thus, if there is an $=$ sign in the statement, the machine will place the result of the calculation of the terms to the right of the $=$ sign in the location symbolized to the left of the $=$ sign. All kinds of bookkeeping information will have to be performed, such as finding a space in memory for every variable in the program.

The procedure may be very complex, with hierarchies of orders upon orders, but the control unit carries out the orders rapidly, accurately, and dependably.

ARITHMETIC

The arithmetic–logic unit of the machine performs all the calculations, by adding binary numbers two at a time, under the command of the control unit, itself under the control of the steps in the program. The arithmetic unit is a binary adder. The addition of $1 + 1$ on this unit is not 2, it is 0 carry 1. Each location on the adder is a flip-flop (an electronic circuit which can read either 0 or 1). That is, it can either send a signal or not; and every time it is pulsed, it changes from 1 to 0 or vice versa. By means of this maneuver the digital computer can outcompute the best mathematician or accountant. It can perform roughly $1\frac{1}{2}$ million calculations in 1 second (if the calculation is simple binary addition). Its multiplication speed is one hundred-fold less, i.e., 150,000 multiplications in 1 second.

STORAGE

The key to the modern digital computer is the stored program concept, developed by John von Neumann with an assist from Norbert

Wiener. The latter conceived the idea from its analogy to the human brain, using cybernetics. We are all stored program machines; and computers can store information just as we do. We are adaptive, however, because we can change our program to adapt to problems in the environment. When computers are made to do this, we say that they are heuristic. We write a program for the computer to cover every contingency that it is possible to predict.

The working storage unit is a configuration of iron-ferrite toroids, located in three dimensions by their x-y-z coordinates. Thus, core 1-2-3 is located by the coordinates (1,2,3) for (x,y,z). When core 1-2-3 is magnetized, the digit 1 is stored at that point. When it is not magnetized, the digit 0 is stored at that point. All the cores of the working memory are scanned at the "read rate" of the computer. Thus, if the computer has a 1 microsecond access time, it reads its entire core memory in 1 microsecond. All information is stored in binary numbers in the core unit. When it is brought out for use elsewhere, however, it is stored in a register, which contains a set of permanent circuits called "flip-flops."

The flip-flop may also have only two positions, corresponding to the zero or one position. Every time a pulse enters a flip-flop, it changes its stored digit. Thus, if a zero is stored in the flip-flop, the next pulse changes it to a 1. If the computer is specified as a 16-bit machine, it will have 16 flip-flops in each register to store the 16 pulses of each computer word.

In addition to the core memory which is the on-line workhorse, there are other forms of memory available for the computer. The disk memory is called the disk file. It consists of a plastic wafer or plate coated with magnetic powder, on each side of which 500,000 words of data can be recorded and stored. Reading and writing are done with a noncontacting head precisely positioned over the disk. Instead of the spiral of phonograph records, the disk file possesses concentric circles with the same number of points on each circle. They are closer together on the smaller diameter and farther apart on the larger diameter. The computer can locate any position on the plastic plate by moving the head to, say, position 1231 in circle 12. The plate rotates continually and is read on the move. Since the logic of the computer can match a spot in 850 nanoseconds to 4 microseconds, the error in location is not very large.

If a twelve-inch circle were moving at 1800 rpm (30 revolutions per second), twelve inches would revolve in $1/30$ of a second or one inch in $1/360$ of a second, or 0.001 inch in 4 microseconds.

Information stored on the disk is usually read sequentially into the core memory, so that only the first piece of information needs to be located; the rest is read in bulk.

Larger capacity bulk storage is furnished by the magnetic tape in which social security records are stored, and located in sufficient time to be useful for payroll calculations. The magnetic tape is again cued to the first position and then bulk transferred to the disk or to the core memory for use in the computer calculations.

LOGIC

The logic unit is a circuit that can perform binary logic of the AND-OR-NOT type. Binary logic is derived from Boolean algebra, developed by George Boole in 1847, long before computers existed. A Boolean AND means that the effect is present only if both conditions are present. It is equivalent to the sign X for

$$1 \times 1 = 1, \quad \text{if A and B, then 1}$$
$$1 \times 0 = 0, \quad \text{if A and not B, then 0}$$
$$0 \times 1 = 0, \quad \text{if not A and B, then 0}$$
$$0 \times 0 = 0, \quad \text{if not A and not B, then 0}$$

A Boolean OR is equivalent to the sign + for

$$1 + 1 = 1, \quad \text{if A or B, then 1}$$
$$1 + 0 = 1, \quad \text{since either A or B is present}$$
$$0 + 1 = 1, \quad \text{since either A or B is present}$$
$$0 + 0 = 0, \quad \text{since neither A nor B is present}$$

A Boolean NOT refers to the other member of the binary team. NOT 1 is 0; NOT 0 is 1. A very interesting algorithm arises between AND-OR-NOT

$$\text{NOT A AND NOT B} = \text{NOT (A OR B)}$$

This can be demonstrated by a principle known as DeMorgan's theorem, using *rich* and *poor*, and *man* and *woman*.

$$\text{If R} = \text{rich} \quad \overline{\text{R}} = \text{not rich} = \text{poor}$$
$$\text{If M} = \text{man} \quad \overline{\text{M}} = \text{not man} = \text{woman}$$

Note that

$$\overline{\text{RM}} = \text{not (rich and man)}$$

could be

$$\text{rich and not man} = \text{rich woman}$$

or

$$\text{man and not rich} = \text{poor man}$$

and $\overline{\text{R}} + \overline{\text{M}} = $ not rich or not man would be poor woman. Hence,

$$\overline{\text{RM}} = \overline{\text{R}} + \overline{\text{M}}$$

Not a rich man = poor woman.

APPLICATIONS OF DIGITAL COMPUTERS

Our primary concern in this discussion is to show how digital computers can be used for biomedical applications. Several papers presented at the Eighth and Ninth ISA Biomedical Sciences Instrumentation Conferences (1970–1971) describe applications of digital, analog, or hybrid computers.

One of the important diagnostic studies of heart performance is the angiograph. A radiopaque dye is introduced into the heart by a catheter, and its progress through the heart chambers is followed on the fluoroscope. The change with time of left ventricular volume is important. A motion picture camera record of the fluoroscopic examination is viewed frame by frame to obtain this information (Trenholm et al., 1970). A television-computer interface which translates the data into computer language is used. A flying spot scans the video information and converts it into digital information, which may be recorded together with relevant physiologic data for future use.

An automatic system to regulate the carbon dioxide inspired by the patient, and subsequent computer handling of the data have proved useful in studying the respiratory control system in man. The carbon dioxide in the inhaled air is programmed by the digital computer to follow any program required by the experimenter—sinusoidal, step, and saw-tooth signals have been employed. The physiologic output is monitored by a special purpose analog computer which calculates and displays the experimental variables in real time and converts them to digital signals which can be stored and processed by the digital computer (Swanson, 1970).

The measurement of the blood pressure of a patient in an Intensive Care Unit is by an invasive technique, i.e., a catheter is inserted into the blood vessel to provide the pressure source for the transducer. Lee and Lewis (1971) describe a noninvasive technique which is made possible by a digital computer. A standard blood pressure cuff is inflated automatically under the control of the computer. The pressure in the cuff and the sounds of the blood vessels under the cuff are converted to digital information by a pressure module and a microphone respectively, both with analog-to-digital converters. The computer also monitors the ECG, electrical impedance of the thorax, and the temperature, and displays the information on a cathode ray tube.

A state-wide communications network under computer control is described by Stratbucker and Chambers (1971) for the state of Nebraska. Improved emergency medical care for victims of traffic accidents can be obtained if information concerning the patient is radioed to the hospital while the victim is being transported there. Sensors in the ambulance detect the patient's vital signs such as heart rate, blood pressure, respiration rate, and peripheral blood flow.

These signals are transmitted to a physician on duty at the hospital who, anticipating the patient's arrival, prepares emergency equipment, and radios back to the ambulance emergency procedures to be conducted en route.

The computer monitors and stores information from the ambulance. In response to a 483 Hz. tone, the computer sends an answering signal advising the ambulance that the information is being recorded and activates a four-channel demodulator to record the data. During transmission, the computer acknowledges receipt of data by periodically sending back signals, and at the end of transmission disconnects the receiver and displays an analysis of the data received for action by the attending physician.

The University of Missouri has undertaken a field demonstration of automatic health care in a rural area by installing a medical information system in a physician's office in Salem, Missouri, and processing the information in a computer located at the campus in Columbia, Missouri (Miller, Adams, and Simons, 1971). The program demonstrates the numerous principles developed in this discussion for an "automated physician's assistant," which collects all the information required by the physician on each patient who visits his clinic, stores the information in a computer file, and presents a summary file to the physician in the form desired. Blood samples and X-ray films are carried by messenger to the clinical laboratory and to the X-ray diagnostic center from whence the results are transmitted to the computer by a remote terminal.

Of interest and as a summary of the possibilities of biomedical instrumentation in the automation of health care are the various parts of the "automated" physical examination performed by this computer system at the physician's request. Procedures described include 1) automated case history, 2) automated chemical laboratory tests, 3) automated ECG analysis, 4) recording and analysis of the physical examination by nurse and doctor, 5) automated blood pressure analysis, 6) hearing test—conducted by the automatic recording audiometer, 7) vision test—conducted by the nurse (results are entered in the patient's file), 8) analysis of X-ray film by a radiologist (results are entered through a remote console into the patient's file), 9) review by the physician of all the information in the patient's file as summarized by the computer (his comments include diagnosis, request for additional tests, management of the patient on subsequent office visits, recommendations for hospitalization), 10) forwarding of complete file to the hospital where it becomes part of the hospital records.

SUMMARY

In systems engineering, engineering techniques are applied to the development of systems, and systems techniques are applied to the engineering of biomedical projects. Systems techniques were introduced in Chapter 1 (block diagram) and have been used to define operational organization throughout the text. In the present chapter the two modern tools of systems engineering, the analog computer and the digital computer, were introduced. The analog computer uses operational amplifiers to construct an electronic analog of a system, which can be tested and manipulated to define its static and dynamic properties.

The function of the digital computer is to interpret large quantities of data. It can monitor and record patient information, symptoms, ECG's, and EEG's. It can compute complex respiratory information to help in the diagnosis of respiratory disease. It can be used to control the flow of information, the administration of complex drugs, or the radiation treatment of breast cancer. It can also be used to simulate complex systems or even analog systems, by using numerical analysis to solve differential equations.

EXERCISES

1. Write an initiation report for a "black box" that will diagnose normal and abnormal heart conditions from an I lead ECG.

2. Write an initiation report for a multiphasic screening center that will diagnose all the abnormal conditions referred to in this chapter.

3. Write an initiation report for a digital computer program that scans chest X-rays and is used in the diagnosis of lung disease.

4. Write an organization report for a systems engineering study to develop a tool for the diagnosis of respiratory diseases like asthma, bronchitis, and emphysema.

5. For the preliminary design, specify and list all equipment required to use a computer monitoring system for patient monitoring in a large metropolitan hospital.

6. Draw a complete analog computer flow diagram for the circulatory system discussed under "Computer Systems."

7. Draw an analog simulation flow diagram for the breathing cycle based on resistance of the airways, R, and compliance of the lung tissue, C.

8. When the human body is subjected to intense, prolonged, or selected frequencies of vibration, some of the organs are displaced from their natural position and permanently damaged. Develop an analog computer simulation to study the susceptibility of an organ such as the liver, the lungs, the heart, or the spleen to be shaken loose from its "moorings" when subjected to vibrations of different intensity, frequency, or duration.

9. Develop a digital computer block diagram to apply logic to the signals emanating from a patient in a coronary care ward bedside unit, to detect potential hazards to the patient.

10. Outline the phases in a systems engineering project connected with the design and construction of a multiphasic screening center, using all the techniques outlined in this chapter, to which any citizen could go to be screened for disease.

General Literature Cited and References

Ashley, J. R. Introduction to Analog Computation. New York: Wiley, 1963.

Bartee, T. C. Digital Computer Fundamentals. New York: McGraw-Hill, 1960.

Blesser, W. B. A Systems Approach to Biomedicine. New York: McGraw-Hill, 1969.

Brown, J. H. U., Jacobs, J. E., and Stark, L. Biomedical Engineering. Philadelphia: Davis, 1971.

Chestnut, H. Systems Engineering Methods. New York: Wiley, 1967.

Goode, H. H., and Machol, R. E. System Engineering. New York: McGraw-Hill, 1957.

Lee, B., and Lewis, F. J. Monitoring of blood pressure of patients in an intensive care unit by a noninvasive technique employing a digital computer and an electropneumatic converter. *Biomed. Sci. Instrumentation 8*, 61: 1971.

Martin, F. F. Computer Modeling and Simulation. New York: Wiley, 1968.

Miller, O. W., Adams, G. E., and Simmons, E. M. Assessing the potential of automated health care in a rural area. *Biomed. Sci. Instrumentation 8,* 19:1971.

Spencer, D. D. The Computer Programmer's Dictionary and Handbook. Waltham, Mass.: Blaisdell, 1968.

Stratbucker, R. A., and Chambers, W. A. Vital function telemetry as part of a mobile emergency medical care system. *Biomed. Sci. Instrumentation 8,* 6:1971.

Swanson, G. D., Snider, D. E., Carpenter, T. M., and Bellville, J. W. A hybrid computer system for on-line respiratory studies. *Biomed. Sci. Instrumentation 7,* 4:1970.

Trenholm, B. G., Winter, D. A., and Dinn, D. F. Digital computer analysis of left ventricular volume from videoangiograms. *Biomed. Sci. Instrumentation 7,* 1:1970.

Wilson, I. G., and Wilson, M. E. Information, Computers and Systems Design. New York: Wiley, 1965.

Glossary

ACCEPTOR. A trivalent element such as indium or gallium, which is added in small concentration to a tetravalent element to provide sites for acceptance of electrons, leaving holes in the tetravalent element.

ACCURACY. The error in a measurement caused by deviation from the true value (as used, it really means inaccuracy). The *percent accuracy* of a measurement is the percent inaccuracy of that measurement, and should be expressed in terms of standard deviation of the measurement. For example, a thermometer with an accuracy of 3% means that a reading of 100°F is $100° \pm (0.03)(100) = 100 \pm 3°F$.

ACTIVE ELEMENT. An energy source in an electrical circuit, voltage, or current source; or an element which contains a voltage or current source, e.g., a vacuum tube or transistor which contains a dependent active source.

ADENOSINE DIPHOSPHATE (ADP). An ester of adenosine and phosphoric acid which can be oxidized to adenosine triphosphate (ATP), the energy source of the cell. ADP is produced from ATP after energy is released and accumulates the oxygen debt of a muscle, i.e., oxygen is required for the reconversion of ADP to ATP.

ADENOSINE TRIPHOSPHATE (ATP). An ester of adenosine and triphosphoric acid, which serves as the energy source for physiologic processes, especially muscle contraction. It is reduced to ADP during the process.

AMPLIFIER. A device for increasing the magnitude of an input signal. Electronic amplifiers use tubes or transistors; pneumatic amplifiers use nozzle-flapper circuits; hydraulic amplifiers use pistons and fluid pressure.

ANTIDIURETIC HORMONE (ADH). The hormone secreted by the hypothalamus which controls the resorption of water in the kidneys, and hence the fluid concentration in the body.

ARTIFACT. A false signal, used in physiology. Instruments often register noise which simulate a signal. Muscle signals produced when the patient moves will produce an artifact ECG. Artifacts are false signals that look like the real signal.

ATRIAL FIBRILLATION. Irregular and rapid contractions of the atrium independent of the ventricles. Occurs in late stages of heart disease when the damaged cardiac muscle has been strained.

BRADYCARDIA. A form of arrhythmia in which the heart beat is slower than normal (a rate below 60 beats per minute in an adult).

BRIDGE CIRCUIT. A four-arm network by which an unknown resistance, capacitance, inductance, or impedance in one arm can be measured by adjusting the other three arms until the bridge is balanced, and then calculating the unknown value from the three known values.

CAPACITANCE. The change in quantity of a stored energy per unit change in potential. It is a lumped parameter in an electrical circuit, or the compliance of an organic vessel, such as a lung or blood vessel.

CATHODE. That part of the electron tube that generates electrons. In electrochemistry, the electrode that attracts negative ions. A cathode ray tube contains a stream of electrons generated by the cathode or "electron gun," which activates a fluorescent coating on a glass screen to make visible the dynamic progress of an electrical signal.

CENTROSOME. A minute body in the cell believed to be the center of activity during mitosis (cellular division).

CEREBRAL CORTEX. The thin outer layer of the brain consisting of cell bodies of neurons which govern the sensory and motor activities of the brain.

CHEMORECEPTORS. Physiologic receptors which respond to the chemical conditions of the body, such as oxygen concentration, carbon dioxide, and pH of the blood.

COLORIMETER. An instrument of chemical analysis that responds to the color of a sample in the visible region of the spectrum. A light is passed through the sample with specific frequencies selected by color filters. A photocell or phototube is usually used to detect the signal emerging from the sample.

CYBERNETICS. The study of communication and control in animal and machine systems with a view to applying the principles learned in one field to the other.

DECADE. A group, set, or series of ten. A decade box is used to measure resistance; each dial has ten positions, and the minimum sensitivity of each dial is ten times that of the previous dial.

DEOXYRIBONUCLEIC ACID (DNA). An acid found in the nucleus of the cell which is believed to carry the genetic properties of the cell.

DERIVED STANDARD. Measurement standards derived from the three primary variables of mass, length, and time; for example, the standard of velocity derives from length and time standards.

DIASTOLIC. The period in the heart cycle when the heart relaxes and becomes filled with blood (first the atria and then the ventricles). The beginning of the systole completes the filling of the ventricles and closes the mitral valves so that additional contraction of the ventricles can send the blood through the body and lungs.

DIELECTRIC CONSTANT. The ability of a given material to store electrical energy when used between the plates of a capacitor. It is numerically equal to the ratio of the capacitance between a pair of plates with the subject materials, to the capacitance in vacuum of the same pair of plates.

DIFFRACTION. The interference pattern that results when electromagnetic energy passes through a slit. A diffraction grating consists of a series of very fine slits, or parallel reflecting surfaces, which disperses the light into wavelengths in a spectroscope, or spectrometer. A crystal acts like a diffraction grating in an X-ray spectrometer.

DIODE. A two element vacuum tube, or solid state device which can transmit a signal only in one direction.

DONOR. A pentavalent element such as arsenic, which is added to a tetravalent element such as silicon or germanium, to provide sites which have excess charge which can diffuse through the semiconductor and carry a current.

DOPPLER FLOW METER. An ultrasonic flow meter which utilizes the change in frequency with flow produced by the Doppler effect to measure the flow.

ECTOPIC FOCI. The origin of a beat at an abnormal position on the heart. Ectopic beats are abnormal beats that do not fall into the normal rhythm of the heart, because they do not originate at the S-A node (pacemaker) of the heart.

ELECTROMAGNETIC SPECTRUM. Waves that set up alternating electric and magnetic fields at right angles to each other. The spectrum includes radio waves, micro waves, and infrared rays, visible light rays, ultraviolet rays, X-rays, gamma rays, and cosmic rays. These types of radiation have the properties of diffraction, reflection, refraction, interference, and polarization. Analyzers have been built in every region of the spectrum to examine matter by interaction with the energy-absorbing constituents in the atoms, molecules, and crystals of material substances.

ELECTRON TUBE. See Vacuum Tube.

ENDOPLASMIC RETICULUM. A series of canals in the cytoplasm of the cell which contains the enzymes that perform the chemical syntheses of the cell.

FEEDBACK CONTROL. The use of the feedback principle to control a process. A selected variable from the process is measured and compared with a reference value and, based on the difference, action is taken to bring the variable to its reference value.

GRID. That part of the electron tube that controls the flow of electrons from the cathode to the plate.

HENRY. The unit of electrical inductance equal to the inductance of a circuit in which a change in current of one ampere per second produces an induced electromotive force of one volt. The usual unit is the millihenry, which is 1/1000th of a Henry.

HOMEOSTASIS. The feedback mechanism used by living systems to control their internal variables.

IMPEDANCE. A vector representation of the passive, energy-absorbing properties of a circuit. It includes the effect of the inductive and capacitive reactances in a circuit, which are frequency dependent.

INDUCTANCE. The property of a coil to store electrical energy in a magnetic field when current through the coil changes.

INTERNATIONAL STANDARDS. Standards adopted internationally for the volt, ohm, and temperature scale against which government laboratories calibrate their standards.

ISCHEMIA. Obstruction of the circulation to a part of the body, which causes local depletion of oxygen supply to the tissue.

KIRCHHOFF'S LAWS. Kirchhoff's current law states that the algebraic sum of the currents flowing into any node of a circuit is zero. Kirchhoff's voltage law states that the algebraic sum of the voltages around any loop in a network is zero. Together they supply the fundamental tools for the analysis of electrical networks.

LINEAR POTENTIOMETER. A transducer which converts a linear displacement to a proportional change in resistance. It consists of a wound resistance traversed by a linear slider.

LUMPED PARAMETERS. The concentration of a distributed property into a single point for analysis purposes, for example, resistance, capacitance, and inductance.

LINEARLY VARIABLE DIFFERENTIAL TRANSFORMER (LVDT). A transformer with a movable core, which can be displaced between coils so that the voltage output of the transformer is proportional to the linear displacement of the core.

MAGNETIC FLOW METER. A flow-measuring device consisting of a magnetic field generator and a pair of electrodes perpendicular to that field. The field is generated across a flowing conductive liquid which generates a voltage proportional to its flow rate.

MICROELECTRODE. An electrode constructed of hollow, drawn capillary glass tubing filled with dilute potassium chloride solution, with a tip approximately 1 micron in diameter so that it can penetrate the membrane of a living cell and measure the intracellular potential.

MITOCHONDRION. An organelle or small organ within the cell whose function is to carry out the metabolic functions of the cell. It is the powerhouse of the cell.

MITOSIS. Normal cell division in which each chromosome separates into two parts and becomes a part of the nucleus of the new cells.

MONOCHROMATIC. Said of light or electromagnetic radiation when the entire signal is of the same frequency or wavelength. It is produced by a monochromator by the diffraction of electromagnetic energy into its component spectrum.

MYOCARDIAL INFARCTION. A portion of the heart musculature that suffers necrosis owing to lack of oxygen supply when a coronary blood vessel is obstructed.

NUCLEUS OF ATOM. The positively charged center of the atom consisting of neutrons and protons and containing most of the mass of the atom.

NUCLEUS OF CELL. A mass of protoplasm in the center of the cell contain-

ing the essential elements that control the growth, metabolism, and reproduction of the cell (now believed to be concentrated in the DNA), and
carried to the cytoplasm of the cell for implementation by ribonucleic acid.

ORGANELLE. An internal organ of the cell, such as the mitochondria or
the endoplasmic reticulum.

OSMOSIS. The process by which a solvent passes through a membrane from
a region of lower solute concentration to a region of higher solute concentration. The tendency of the solvent to pass through the membrane is called
its osmotic pressure.

PASSIVE ELEMENT. An element in a circuit (resistor, capacitor, or inductor), which consumes electrical energy.

PHASE ANGLE. The angle between the vectors representing two signals, for
example, the input and output signals of a transducer or circuit. It can be
measured by projecting the input and output signals as sine waves on an
oscilloscope or recorder, and measuring the distance between corresponding points of the cycle, as a ratio of the total cycle distance of the input
signal.

PHOTOELECTRIC. When radiation impinges on a photoelectric surface,
electrons are emitted from that surface. This principle is used in the photocell and in the photocathode of the phototube, photometers, spectrophotometers, and other electromagnetic analytical instrumentation.

PHOTOMETER. A chemical transducer for the analysis of solutions which
absorb at specific frequencies of the electromagnetic spectrum. The
sample is placed in a cuvette (glass or quartz container) between a radiation
source and a phototube, photocell, or other photosensitive element, and the
amount of absorption at specific frequency ranges selected by optical filters
is measured.

PLATE. That element of the electron tube that attracts the electrons that are
emitted by the cathode and pass through the grid of the tube.

POTENTIOMETER. The term has a dual meaning. One meaning is to "meter
potential," i.e., a slide wire is activated by a known potential across its
total length so that the potential tapped from part of the wire is proportional to the total potential and may be "metered" to a voltage bridge. A
rheostat wired to meter potential is called a "pot" or potentiometer. The
instrument that measures potential is called a potentiometer.

PRECISION. The root-mean-square deviation obtained when the same
measurement is replicated (repeatedly performed in an identical manner).

PRIMARY STANDARD. A standard of mass, length, or time, used as a
reference to establish the accuracy of secondary or derived standards. It
can be the primary standard at the National Bureau of Standards (NBS)
laboratory in Washington, or the primary standard of a local standards
laboratory of an industrial company or military area.

RC NETWORK. When a resistance and capacitance are connected in series
and a voltage used to charge the capacitor, the time-dependent properties
of the current flow approximate many physical, mechanical and biological
phenomena, which are called "first order" because they can be represented
by a first-order differential equation. They are "exponential" because the
solution of the differential equation contains an exponential of the form e^{at}.

They are "time constant" processes because $a = \dfrac{1}{RC}$ where RC is the time constant of the process.

REPLICATION. The repetition of a set of measurements with the same instrument to determine the precision of the measurement.

RESISTANCE. The ratio of potential change to current change produced in a passive element such as a resistor.

SECONDARY MODIFIER. That part of the transducer which converts the sensed signal to an electrical signal.

SECONDARY STANDARD. A standard provided by the NBS for local laboratories to use in the calibration of their primary standards.

SENSITIVITY. The change in reading of an instrument per unit change in the measured variable, for example, millimeter of scale per square inch change in pressure.

SENSOR. That part of a transducer that senses the variable and converts it to a (usually) mechanical displacement or force.

SERVOMECHANISM. An electronic control system in which a low energy electrical signal supplies a high energy output to move a mechanical mechanism, such as a chart drive, or rudder of a boat.

SERVOMOTOR. A feedback controlled motor, usually electrical or hydraulic, in which the output of a system is compared with a reference value, and the difference between these signals drives the motor in a direction so that the difference tends to disappear.

SERVOSYSTEM. A system in which servomechanisms augment a measurement to produce a useful mechanical output.

SPECTROGRAPH. An instrument used to record an electromagnetic spectrum, usually photographically, generated by an incandescent specimen. The specimen may be made incandescent by an arc or flame, its radiation is diffracted by a prism or grating, and the diffracted lines are recorded by exposure to a photographic film. Spectrographs are also used for studies of stars and the sun.

SPECTROMETER. An instrument used to measure the intensity of each wavelength of an electromagnetic spectrum transmitted by a gas or liquid specimen or (for an X-ray spectrometer) a solid specimen. Typical spectrometers include gamma ray, X-ray, and mass spectrometers. The mass spectrometer causes dispersion of the mass numbers of an ionized specimen and measures the intensity of each of the masses.

SPHYGMOMANOMETER. The blood pressure measuring cuff.

STANDARD OF MEASUREMENT. A carefully calibrated measurement which can be used to establish the accuracy of other measurements. See also Primary, Secondary, International, and Derived Standards.

STENOSIS. Constriction of a flow passage in the body. Cardiac stenosis appears in the heart when any of the flow passages in the heart are constricted by scar tissue. Mitral stenosis, the result of rheumatic heart disease, is a constriction of the mitral valve between the left atrium and the left ventricle of the heart.

STRAIN GAUGE. A transducer that changes in resistance with a change in applied strain. It is used for measuring displacement and force as well as strain by being mounted on an elastic element which produces strain from displacement or force.

SYSTOLIC. The active portion of the heart cycle in which the heart is contracting, and blood is being pumped out of the chambers of the heart.

TACHYCARDIA. An abnormal heart rate in which the heart is beating more rapidly than normal (usually applied to a heart rate in excess of 100 beats per minute).

THERMISTOR. A temperature transducer containing a metal oxide mixture whose resistance decreases with temperature.

THERMOCOUPLE. A temperature transducer consisting of a junction of dissimilar materials, for example, two metals, that produces a voltage proportional to its temperature.

THERMOGRAPHY. The technique of measuring body surface temperature by means of a radiation detector in order to detect physiologic abnormalities, breast cancer, for example.

TRANSDUCER. A device for converting a measurement to a more useful signal, for example, a pressure transducer converts a pressure measurement to a displacement which can be readily converted to an electrical or pneumatic signal. The transducer consists of a primary sensor, a secondary modifier, and an output element.

TRANSISTOR. Two diodes that when hooked back-to-back furnish a conducting path which can be modulated by a signal to the base or common element. The transistor has three elements (emitter, collector, and base). It can have NPN or PNP configuration, where N is negative and P is positive.

TRANSMITTANCE. The ratio of light flux transmitted by a medium to the light flux incident on it. The absorbance of a sample is proportional to the logarithm of the transmittance. The concentration of a component in the sample is proportional to the absorbance.

TRANSMITTER. The output element of a transducer which is capable of transmitting a signal proportional to the original sensed variable to a remote display element.

TRIODE. A three-element vacuum tube containing a grid, cathode, and plate, and capable of amplifying signals by having the grid modulate the current between the cathode and plate.

ULTRASONIC FLOW METER. A transducer which uses a piezoelectric crystal to generate and detect the ultrasonic signal sent across a flow channel. The signal obtained is proportional to the flow of the fluid through the channel. See *Doppler Flow Meter.*

VACUUM TUBE. A glass tube containing electron-generating and electron-receiving elements in an evacuated container. Parts of the tube are the cathode, plate, and grid.

VARIABLE INDUCTANCE TRANSDUCER. A transducer that measures displacement by causing the displacement to move an element in a magnetic circuit which changes its inductance.

VARIABLE RELUCTANCE TRANSDUCER. A transducer which measures displacement by having the displacement move an element in a magnetic circuit which changes its reluctance.

VENTRICULAR FIBRILLATION. Rapid, incomplete contractions of the ventricle of the heart. They may be produced by electrical shock or by blockage in the coronary vessels of the heart.

WAVELENGTH. In a periodic wave, the distance between points of corresponding phase of two consecutive cycles. The wavelength of an electromagnetic wave times the frequency is equal to the velocity of light, 3×10^{10} cm. per second.

WHEATSTONE BRIDGE. A four-arm bridge used for measuring resistance. Three of the four arms are known resistances, one of which is usually adjustable. The value of the unknown resistance in the fourth arm can be calculated from the known resistances, $R_x = R_{adj} \times \dfrac{R_1}{R_2}$.

ZENER DIODE EFFECT. Results from trying to pass a back current through a diode. The reverse current is constant and is used as a DC reference current in modern instrumentation.

Collateral Reading

The greater portion of the current literature in Biomedical Instrumentation can be found in

BIOMEDICAL SCIENCES INSTRUMENTATION, Vols. 1– (1963–),
   published by Instrument Society of America, Pittsburgh, Penna.
ANNUAL PROCEEDINGS of the International Conference on Medical and
   Biological Engineering (Abstracts)
ANNUAL PROCEEDINGS of the Annual Conference on Engineering in
   Medicine and Biology (Abstracts)

and ANNUAL MEETINGS of

American Institute of Chemical Engineers
   345 E. 47 Street, New York, N.Y. 10017
American Society of Mechanical Engineers
   345 E. 47 Street, New York, N.Y. 10017
Association for the Advancement of Medical Instrumentation
   9650 Rockville Pike, Bethesda, Maryland 20014
Institute of Electrical and Electronics Engineers
   345 E. 47 Street, New York, N.Y. 10017
Instrument Society of America
   530 William Penn Place, Pittsburgh, Penna. 15219

References from the first five chapters are to basic information in the specific fields. References in Chapters 6 to 10 are to the above publications.

Index

Absorbance, 146
Acceptor, 269
Accuracy, 5, 6, 269
Acid-base
  buffering action, 110
  control, 108
Action potential, 81
Active circuit element, 16, 24, 269
  transistor, 32
  vacuum tube, 16
Activity coefficient, 117
Adaptive control, 82
Adenosine diphosphate (ADP), 3, 81–82, 269
Adenosine triphosphate (ATP), 3, 81–82, 269
Adrenocorticotropic hormone (ACTH), 108
Adsorption chromatography, 171
Aging, EEG estimation of, 205
Airway resistance, 221
Alarm instrumentation, 15, 188, 190
Aldosterone, 106
Alpha brain waves, 85, 202, 203
  radiation, 63
Alternating bridges, 72, 125
Alternating current (AC), 20
Amino acid analysis, 170
  buffer, 110
Ammeter, 39
Amplification factor, 16
Amplifier, 15, 33, 269
  operational, 37–38; transistor, 35–36; vacuum tube, 33–34
Amplitude modulation (AM), 234
Analog computer, 251
Analyzers, 9
  automatic, 230, 231; bedside, 150; blood, 230; cadmium, 132; calcium, 133; carbon dioxide, 231; chloride, 130; clinical, 229–232, 265; colorimetric, 146–147; conductivity, 122; infrared, 155; oxygen, 129, 231; pH, 122, 231; photometer, 147, 273; polarographic, 126; potassium ion, 133; potentiometric, 118; quadrupole resonance, 162; serum, 133; sodium ion, 130; specific ion, 129; spectral emission, 156; spectrophotometer, 149; ultraviolet, 146; x-ray, 163–166
Anemia, 215
Anesthesia, 203
Angiograph, automated, 264
Antidiuretic hormone (ADH), 3, 108, 269
Arrhythmia, 189

bradycardia, 185, 270; monitor, 189; tachycardia, 185, 275
Artifact, 270
Asthma, 221
Atom, structure of, 141–143
Atomic absorption, 159
Atrial fibrillation, 186, 270
Atrial-ventricular (AV) shunt, 215
Autocorrelation function, 204
Automated health care, 265
Automatic blood analyzers, 64, 230
Automation, anesthetic, 264, 265; angiographic, 264; blood analysis, 230; blood pressure cuff, 265; carbon dioxide analysis in, 231; carbon dioxide control in, 264; clinical laboratory tests, 229, 265; digital logging, 232; emergency medical network 265; health care, 265; oxygen analysis, 231; pH analysis, 231; physicians' case history, 265; respiratory function test, 264
Autonomic nervous system (ANS), 84

Ballistocardiograph, 217
Bedside monitor, 188
  analyzer requirements, 150; arrhythmia, 189; blood pressure, 178, 188; heart rate, 181, 188; pulse rate, 181, 188; respiration rate, 180, 188; temperature, 176, 188
Beer-Lambert law, 144–146
Beta brain waves, 86, 202, 203
  radiation, 63
Bicarbonate buffer, 110
Biological sensors, 86
Biological sensory nerve endings (table), 87
Biological systems, 10
  analysis, 10
    capillary system, 103
    cell, 78–82
      energy, 81; memory, 82; power production, 81; signal transmission, 79
    circulatory system, 87–95; fluid volume, 101; kidneys, 104; lymphatic system, 103; nervous system, 82–86; respiratory system, 95
  control, 82
    acid-base, 108–110; blood pressure, 91; body fluid, 101; breathing, 99; chemical composition, 106; cogitation, 85; fluid control, 107; homeo-

Feedback control, 2, 271. See also *Control*.
ANS and, 84; block diagram of, 83;
blood composition and, 84; pressure,
84, 91–92; canonical form of, 12, 83;
definition of, 12; homeostasis and, 84,
271; nervous system and, 82; on-off
control and, 83, 84; peristalsis and, 83;
reflexive control as, 83; regulation of,
84; servocontrol as, 83, 274; temperature in, 84
Fetal head visualization, 211
Fibrillation, heart, 186
Fick method, 215
Filtration, kidney, 105
"Finger print" method, 148
Fixed rate pacemaker, 239
Flame photometry, 159
Flapper nozzle, 55
Flow measurement, 62–63
differential pressure and, 62; magnetic,
62, 272; orifice in, 62; renal blood,
225; ultrasonic, 62–63, 213–214, 275
Fluid control, 107
extracellular, 102; hypothalamus, 85;
intracellular, 102; osmotic, 101;
plasma, 102
flow, 90
Fluoride ion detection, 131
Force balance recorder, 46
Force measurement, 56
by displacement, 56; by strain gauge,
56, 274
Frequency, definition of.
of light, 272; modulation (FM), 234;
standard, 8
Fugacity, 117
Functional residual air, 217
Functional residual volume, 220

Galvanometer, Einthoven, 186
recorder in, 45; string, 186
Gamma radiation, 63
Gamma ray instruments, 63
Gas chromatograph, 64
Gastrointestinal control, 85
Geiger-Müller counter, 165
Globar, 154
Glycogen, 4
Grand mal epilepsy, 203
Grid, vacuum tube, 33, 271
Guldberg and Waage law, 116
Guyton, cardiac output after, 214

Half-cells, 121
Hays bridge, 75
Head injury, diagnosis of, 211
Hearing test, digital, 265
Heart, 2, 92, 181–183
activity of, 181; atrium of, 92; axis of,
183–185; block, 240; chest electrodes

and, 95; disease, atrial fibrillation as,
270
bradycardia in, 270; coronary blockage as, 275; ectopic foci in, 189, 271;
ischemia in, 272; myocardial infarction as, 186, 215, 272; stenosis in,
207, 274; ventricular fibrillation as,
186, 275
ECG and, 94, 181; electrical properties
of, 181–185; limb leads and, 95; lung
machine, 207; mechanical activity of,
182; murmurs, 93; phonocardiogram
of, 93; rate, 85, 185, 275, 290
arrhythmia of, 189; bradycardia and,
185, 270; hypothalamic control of,
85; monitor of, 181; tachycardia and,
185, 275
sounds, 207; phonocardiographic detection of, 205; stenosis and, 274; ventricle, 92

Impedance, 19–23, 272
capacitive, 23; inductive, 21, 22; measurement of, 73–76, 225; resistive, 20;
vector representation of, 19, 226
Impedance bridges, 73–76
capacitive, 73–74; inductive, 75; plethysmography and, 225–229
Impedance of tissue, 228
calibration of leg and, 228; cardiac, 229;
renal, 228; thoracic, 228
Impedance matching, cathode follower in,
37
operational amplifier in, 38–39; transistor in, 36; vacuum tube in, 37
Impedance plethysmography, 19, 225–229
bipolar bridge and, 225; calibration of
tissue and, 228; cardiac output in,
229; renal blood flow and, 228; thoracic impedance in, 229
Implanted pacemaker, 241
Inductance, 15, 18–19, 272
bridges, 73–74; displacement measurement in, 53; impedance vector, 21,
22; mutual, 18; self, 18
Infrared absorption bands, 152–153
analysis, 151–156; continuous analyzer,
154–156; spectrometer, 153–154;
thermography, 63
Input resistance, 17
Inspiratory capacity (IC), 220
Instrumental methods of analysis, 10
Instrumentation analysis. See *Analyzers*.
bedside, 187; blood pressure, 188; central station, 190; ECG, 183–186; heart
rate, 188; hospital, 192; pulse rate,
188; safety, 192; science, 5
Intercellular fluid volume, 102
Intercellular ionic activity, 133
Intercellular potential, 79–81, 272

tem, 85; sympathetic, 85; synapses, 83
Nessler method, 146
Neurophysiology, 2
N-P-N transistor, 33
Nuclear instrumentation, 168–169
Nucleic acid analysis
Nucleolus, 4
Nucleus, atomic, 141, 272
  cellular, 4, 272

Octave, 208
Ohm, 16
  standard, 7
Ohmic resistance, 17
Operational amplifiers, 37–38, 126, 252
Optical isolation link, 199
Optimizing control, 82
Organelles, 4, 272
  centrosome, 5, 270; endoplasmic reticulum, 271; mitochondrion, 272; nucleolus, 4; nucleus, 4, 272
Orifice flow measurements, 62
Oscillograph, 45
Oscilloscope, 15, 40
  automatic, 44; Lissajous, 44; normal mode, 43; phase angle, 273
Osmoreceptors, 3, 108
Osmosis, 273
  fluid control and, 101–102; membrane transport and, 101; pressure and, 101, 273
Output element, 275
Owen bridge, 75, 76
Oxygen, analysis of, 231
  chemoreceptor and, 270; debt, 3; dissolved, 129; respiration and, 95

Pacemakers, 237–243
  batteries in, 236; demand rate of, 238; electrodes in, 238; external, 239; fixed rate, 242; heart block and, 237; implanted, 241; percutaneous, 240; power source of, 236; pulse generator and, 238; radio-frequency, 241; synchronous, 238; transvenous, 241; types (table), 239
Parathyroid hormone control, 106
Paroxysmal tachycardia, 186
Partial pressure, 95
Passive circuit element, 24, 273
  capacitance of, 26, 270; electrical circuits and, 16; inductance and, 15, 272; resistance and, 274
Patient monitor, 175–200
  bedside, 187–189; central station, 190–192; electrocardiogram and, 181–187; resuscitation and, 189; safety requirements of, 192–199; sensors in, 176–181

heart rate, 181; pressure, 178; pulse rate, 181; respiration, 180; temperature, 176–178
Patient reference ground, 193
Periodic table of elements, 144
Peripheral resistance, 89
Peristalsis, telemetry of, 233
Petit mal epilepsy, 203
Pfund infrared analyzer, 155
pH analysis, 231
  chemoreceptor, 270; measurement, 122
Phase angle, 273
Phases of system engineering, 248–251
  final design, 250; initiation of, 248; organization of, 248; preliminary design, 249; test of, 250–251
Phonocardiography, 205–209
Phosphate buffer, 110
  ion detector, 132
Photocell, barrier type, 147
  in colorimetry, 147; photoelectric emission and, 273
Photographic recorders, 47
Photometer, 147, 273
Photomultiplier, 147
Phototube, in spectrophotometer, 149
Physical examination data storage, 265
Physical measurements, chemical composition and, 10, 137–173
  mechanical, 52–58
Physiology, 2, 78–112
Piezoelectric parameters, displacement measurement and, 55
  flow measurement and, 63, 275; ultrasound and, 209–210
Placenta, localization of, 211
Plasma, 102
Plate, vacuum tube, 33, 273
Platinum resistance thermometer, 8
Platinum thermocouple, 8
P-N junction, 30
P-N-P transistor, 32, 33
Pneumatic displacement measurement, 55
Pneumotachograph, 221
Pneumotaxic reflex, 100
Poiseuille's law, flow resistance and, 88
Polarography, 10, 126–129
  biomedical, 128; Clark cell and, 129; continuous flow in, 129; dissolved oxygen in, 129; dropping mercury electrode (DME) and, 126; Hersch cell in, 129; Heyrovsky and, 126; voltammetry and, 126
Positive filter infrared analyzer, 156
Potassium, in cell, 81
  in ion electrode, 133
Potential in solution, 118–122
  electrodes and, 120–121; half-cell, 121; Nernst equation and, 121; oxidation-